THE COMPLETE
ILLUSTRATED GUIDE TO

TAI CHI

THE COMPLETE ILLUSTRATED GUIDE TO

TAI CHI

A Practical Approach to the
Ancient Chinese Movement for
Health and Well-being

ANGUS CLARK

ELEMENT

Shaftesbury, Dorset • Boston, Massachusetts • Melbourne, Victoria

© Element Books Limited 2000

First published in Great Britain in 2000 by
ELEMENT BOOKS LIMITED
Shaftesbury, Dorset SP7 8BP

Published in the USA in 2000 by
ELEMENT BOOKS INC
160 North Washington Street, Boston MA 02114

Published in Australia in 2000 by
ELEMENT BOOKS LIMITED
and distributed by Penguin Australia Ltd
487 Maroondah Highway, Ringwood, Victoria 3134

Note from the Publisher
Any information given in this book is not intended to be taken
as a replacement for medical advice. Any person with a condition requiring
medical attention should consult a qualified practitioner or therapist.

Designed and created for Element Books with
THE BRIDGEWATER BOOK COMPANY LIMITED

ELEMENT BOOKS LIMITED
Editorial Director: SUE HOOK
Senior Commissioning Editor: CARO NESS
Project Editor: FINNY FOX-DAVIES
Group Production Director: CLARE ARMSTRONG
Production Manager: STEPHANIE RAGGETT
Production Controller: FIONA HARRISON

THE BRIDGEWATER BOOK COMPANY
Art Director: TERRY JEAVONS
Editorial Director: FIONA BIGGS
Managing Editor: ANNE TOWNLEY
Project Editor: LORRAINE TURNER
Art Directors: GLYN BRIDGEWATER, EMILY WILKINSON
Page Make-up: ANGELA ENGLISH
Picture Research: LIZ MOORE
Illustrations: LORRAINE HARRISON, CATHERINE MCINTYRE, GLYN SMITH
Computer-Generated Illustrations: RICHARD CONSTABLE, DEREK LEE
Three-Dimensional Models: MARK JAMIESON
Studio Photography: GUY RYECART

Printed and bound in Great Britain by
Butler & Tanner Ltd

Library of Congress Cataloging in Publication
data available

British Library Cataloguing in Publication data available

ISBN 1 86204 451 1 (Hardback)
ISBN 1 86204 452 X (Paperback)

CONTENTS

1

ORIGINS AND HISTORY

2

A BODY-BASED PRACTICE

3

TAKING STEPS AND MAKING MOVES

THE COMPLETE SHORT FORM

TAI CHI - THE BROADER PICTURE

TAI CHI FOR CREATIVE LIVING

LIFE STORIES

HOW TO USE THE BOOK

The Complete Illustrated Guide to Tai Chi is a comprehensive introduction to an ancient Eastern practice that is becoming more and more popular in the West in response to the pressures of modern life. Many people think of tai chi purely as a system of exercise; in fact it is a holistic healing art which embraces body, mind, and spirit. It improves physical and mental health through posture training and exercising all parts of the body, combined with encouraging greater awareness of the links between body and mind. The result is better health and a sense of well-being. Practiced regularly and with dedication, tai chi becomes a system of self-development, deepens awareness of the self and of other people, and encourages a flowering of personal creativity.

This book is divided into seven parts. Part 1 looks at the history of tai chi, from its roots in Taoist thought to the development of the different schools.

Part 2 examines its impact on the human body and the benefits it can bring.

Clear text explaining each body system and its function

Full color illustrations showing key parts of the body

Detailed information on specific parts of the body

THE POSITIONING OF THE FEET

Both feet on the ground

Right heel off the ground

Right foot off the ground

To help with the stepping in each posture, diagrams are given for the foot positions showing how and where to place the feet and in which direction you should be facing. The dimensions of the "box" represent the feet placed one shoulders-width apart. North is at the bottom. For each posture the box remains fixed and the foot positions move around it – see pages 94–95 Single Whip, where the foot positions move around the fixed box to show the stepping sequence. To indicate whether the foot is on the ground, lifting off it, or clear of the ground the foot positions are colored. Black shows that the foot is placed flat on the ground, gray shows that the heel or toe is lifting up, and the foot outline indicates that the foot is clear of the ground. For example, on page 120 Separate Right Foot, the feet are shown black and in contact with the ground until the right heel is lifted and shows gray in Step 3. The right foot is outlined in Step 4 to show that it is off the ground. In some postures the box will have a slightly different position in order to clearly show the best position for the steps to follow. However, the box does sometimes remain in the same place for consecutive postures.

Part 3 introduces the basic stances and movements, in preparation for Part 4, which takes you step by step through the sequence of movements of the Chen Man-ch'ing Short Form, featuring a short variation introduced by the 20th-century teacher Chi Chiang-tao. The form is performed as an unending sequence of movements which flow from page to page, and this is emphasized in the way the postures are presented photographically.

It is traditional to begin the Tai Chi short form sequence by facing north (see page 63).

To facilitate practice, the body position, orientation and weight distribution are shown at the start of each two-page spread

Main text explains the purpose of the posture in the form

Main text gives comprehensive, easy to follow information

Photographs and drawings illustrate general text

Part 5 explores the partner practice called Pushing Hands, and the major branches of the art, including tai chi weapons practice and qigung (chigung or qi gong).

Parts 6 and 7 consider the role of tai chi in unearthing buried creative abilities and giving them expression.

THE COMPLETE ILLUSTRATED GUIDE TO TAI CHI

PREFACE

Tai chi is a system of exercises or movements to promote health and longevity and a comprehensive system of self-defense. Its roots are in China, where it evolved over many hundreds of years as a martial art and as a system of self-development. In the past, many of its techniques were preserved for generations as clan or family secrets, but very gradually, knowledge of the art spread throughout China. Now at the start and end of every day in villages, towns, and cities all over Chinese Asia, Chinese people can be seen practicing the slow, graceful movements of tai chi in private courtyards and public squares and parks.

Not until the 20th century was tai chi carried to the West, by Westerners who had studied under Chinese masters in Hong Kong or Taiwan, and occasionally on the mainland, and by Chinese teachers who moved to the West. Nowadays, tai chi is well known in all Western countries, and a wide spectrum of people all over the world – women, men, old people, and young who have heard of its benefits – practice it regularly. It is now not uncommon in the West to find health organizations, schools, colleges, and even businesses incorporating it into their curricula and their training programs.

Many people who practice tai chi do so because it adds something special to their lives. What that special something is unfolds for everyone who studies this ancient art. It is my aim in this book to help you on your journey into tai chi, whether you are just taking your first steps or you are already a seasoned traveller.

One early decision students often feel they have to make is whether to practice tai chi for their health alone, or for their health and also to learn a system of self-defense. Many teachers and writers on tai chi categorize the art as one or the other. My approach values tai chi as a system of movement with a variety of health, fighting, and self-development aspects. This book introduces you to all of these. It has sections devoted to healing, the physical body, the subtle body energies of the meridians and energy centers, qigung – a health-orientated practice closely related to tai chi – partner exercises called pushing hands, martial techniques, and weapons forms. Part 6 explores the creative aspects of tai chi and its links with nature. In this way I present tai chi as a multidimensional art form that has the capacity to touch several important levels in the life of anyone who embarks on its exploration. Tai chi is not just about health or about self-defense, but about the development of the whole individual – body, mind, and spirit.

I have also introduced a dimension to the book which further reflects my personal and perhaps unorthodox approach. I use freestyle movement as a way of developing ease of movement and of experiencing the fundamental principles of tai chi – the polarities of yin and yang, explained on pages 18–19. In freestyle movement people are at liberty to move in ways that enable

The snake, in the form of a cascade of cosmic energy, sweeps down from the head to the earth in the posture Squatting Single Whip.

them to experience opposing conditions, such as large and small, or fast and slow, or open and closed. I continually see how this less formal approach gives people greater insight into tai chi and helps them access a deeper experience of the form, as they find they understand more about the energies, forces, and meanings of the body formations or "shapes" created by the postures.

At dawn and as the sun sets in the evening, Chinese people go out to practice tai chi.

I have tried to give as complete a guide to tai chi as is possible in one book. It presents the ideas of sages said to have contributed to tai chi's development in past times, and the writings of modern luminaries of the art, such as Yang Cheng-fu who developed the Yang style Long Form. It recounts the story of tai chi's many styles and schools and gives full step-by-step instructions for performing one internationally known style. The Short Form described on pages 84–143 is the one devised by Cheng Man-ch'ing, a Chinese tai chi teacher who moved to Taiwan, after China's Communist Revolution, with a minor sequence variation added by one of his students, Dr. Chi Ching-tao. Cheng Man-ch'ing and his students spread knowledge of his uniquely soft but powerful form through the East and across to Western countries. In the 1960s Cheng Man-ch'ing moved from Taiwan to New York City, where he opened a school of tai chi. Today his form is practiced worldwide.

The modern world is fast and busy and seems to be getting faster and busier. Personally, culturally, and globally we contend with difficulties and pressures of many different kinds. We can all too easily find ourselves worrying through the day, concerned about some health problem, overwhelmed by pressures of work, or preoccupied by some item from the relentless bombardment of media information. How do we manage such pressure? How do we ensure that our physical, mental, emotional, and spiritual needs are heard and taken care of? Although the roots of tai chi are ancient, I believe that its principles are applicable in a modern world and I hope that you will find answers to these important questions in this book and in your practice of tai chi.

太 11 極

1
ORIGINS AND HISTORY

INTRODUCING TAI CHI

T ai Chi is practical and visionary, technical and magical. It spans the realms of body, mind, and spirit. Practicing every day brings three major benefits: enduring health and a sense of well-being; improved skills in working with other people; and a regular reminder of the human connection to the web of life and to the cosmos.

A single tai chi posture is caught like a frozen frame in a video movie. Although the movements of tai chi are choreographed like a dance and carried out in an unbroken flow, they consist of a sequence of separate postures or poses. This posture is called White Crane Spreads Wings.

Tai chi is a system of movement, exercise, awareness-training, self-development, and martial training suitable for an unusually wide range of people. Although the movements are choreographed and carried out in a set sequence, there is scope for individuals to bring their own physical, mental, and spiritual individuality to the sequence each time they practice.

There are several styles of movement and approaches to tai chi practice (see pages 184–85), some of them historic, some developed in recent years by modern teachers and masters. Each has its distinguishing characteristics and carries the name of the family or clan – Yang, Chen, Wu – through which it evolved. All the principles of tai chi philosophy are put into practice in the non-stop sequence of movements called the form (see pages 84–5), which is the essence of the art. Each tai chi style has its own form or a number of forms which differ from those of other styles in the postures included, the order in which they appear, the way they are performed, and how long they take to run through or play.

Tai chi attracts people of both sexes and all ages, sizes, shapes, intellectual capacity, and emotional and spiritual disposition. Children can benefit from movement based on the principles of tai chi, and everyone from teenagers to mothers to centenarians can practice tai chi and enjoy many of its benefits. There is no point at which people over a certain age, say, are forced to give up, as there is in many sports whose demands can exceed the physical capabilities of men and women as young as 30. Tai chi should become a lifelong activity. It complements the natural processes involved in growing older by helping people of all ages keep the body supple and active, so that it does not degenerate. It provides a steady way of building up solid mental and physical capabilities and developing them for as long as we live.

Practicing tai chi regularly brings a sense of wholeness and well–being, because it stimulates the complicated, interacting system of body and mind. It boosts the blood circulation, for instance, so oxygenating the body's cells, and stimulates vital organs. Generally, tai chi movements increase the mobility of the joints; others stretch and tone muscles, tendons, and ligaments. One sequence of movements realigns the bones of the spine, improving posture. The learning process involves using logic and intuition, so that in time, practice sharpens mental acuity, observation, and concentration. It stimulates the mind as well as the brain, so providing total exercise.

The movements of tai chi are relaxed but precise. They are the physical manifestation of a number of

As well as the solo practice of the form, tai chi may also be carried out with a partner. These exercises are usually called Pushing Hands because they involve pushing and yielding. They provide a socially safe opportunity to experience and explore interpersonal relationships through touch. This is something many Western students find especially valuable.

philosophical principles, carefully worked out and thoughtfully applied. Each posture has its own clear definition, different from that of every other. To be executed correctly it must have the right physical structure. This involves making a particular shape with the whole body, which has a certain effect on the internal organs, the muscles, the ligaments, and the breathing pattern. The posture demands that the attention be focused in a particular way. All these factors combine to create a particular energy field or character for the posture. However free-flowing the movements may appear, it is possible (and necessary)

to account for everything that is happening, physically and mentally, from moment to moment of the practice. To achieve this demands a high level of concentration. With this awareness, however, practice becomes meditation in movement.

Maybe it is something about this primary nature of tai chi that makes it so spellbinding to watch. Although they are essentially down to earth, the purposeful movements of the art unquestionably carry a sense of magic. The slow movements of a figure practicing beneath a tree or framed within a city square always arrest the eye and entrance passers-by.

The shapes and patterns made by our bodies during tai chi practice are the same as those found in nature – the spiral formed by the arms of our galaxy; the way the planets orbit the sun; the movement of a breaking wave; even the pattern newly poured cream makes on the surface of a cup of coffee.

太 15 極

THE ROOTS OF TAI CHI

Tai chi is rooted in the rich soil of ancient Chinese thought, which is based on observing the way things work in nature. The art embodies the concept of continuous change from one extreme to the other as expressed in the ancient book of wisdom, the *I Ching*, "When the sun has reached its meridian, it declines, and when the moon has become full, it wanes." Tai chi stems from the ancient philosophy of Taoism, which arose at a time when China's earliest martial traditions were emerging, among agricultural peoples whose lives were frequently disrupted by wars waged by contending states. And it was founded on the principle of following the natural way or Tao – the ancient philosophy of Taoism.

The origins of tai chi are hidden among the myths and legends of China's ancient history. The first written records of tai chi practice do not appear until the end of the first millennium C.E. However, the art is known to have developed perhaps a thousand years earlier by Taoist recluses who retreated from the world to mountain hermitages where they contemplated the meaning of action by studying nature.

Taoism is an ancient Chinese system of thought which attempts to understand the laws governing change in the universe. By acting in a way that accords with the laws governing change, one might escape entanglement in the evil consequences of change. The Tao or Way is, therefore, the way the universe works, the natural way of things, from the way the clouds form and disperse to the way a person behaves.

The early Taoists in their mountain retreats sought to cultivate the Tao or natural way of being within themselves. They concerned themselves with all aspects of life, from relationships to government to the natural world. They centered their philosophy on the concept of Non-Being. At a government level, this means meddling as little as possible in the workings of the state; and on a personal level it means offering help where it is needed, but never taking an opportunity for self-aggrandisement.

Taoism centers on the concept of effortless action and the power it engenders. Water symbolizes this idea of strength in weakness. It accepts the lowest level without resistance, filling every channel and hollow, yet it wears down the hardest obstacles in its path simply by flowing round them. This knowledge, applied to everyday life, means that striving becomes

The Taoist philosopher Lao Tzu is said to have been Official Archivist of the State of Chou in the first century BCE. When Chou declined, Lao Tzu left. History records that the Keeper of the Pass asked him to set down his knowledge in a book, and he wrote the *Tao Te Ching*.

the antithesis of Taoist action: understanding springs from spontaneous creativity, not from mental or physical effort. Applied to tai chi, it means that struggling to attain a difficult posture is futile. Only union of body and mind – practicing with the right intention behind the movements – ensures success.

Ideas about the Tao or Way and how to follow it must have been evolving for many hundreds of years before they were eventually set down in writing in the *Tao Te Ching (Classic of the Way and Virtue)*, the principal text of Taoism. This small collection of

TAI AND CHI

 In Chinese, the characters for "tai" and "chi" ("tai" and "ji" in modern Chinese spelling, see page 185) express a double superlative, often translated literally as "Supreme Ultimate" or more simply as "cosmos." Tai chi is said to have been born from *wu chi*, the Great Void, the original state of cosmic emptiness. And with the birth of tai chi, stillness changed into movement or energy, nothing into something. This movement was generated by the interplay of the opposing yet complementary forces of yin and yang (see pages 18–19). Tai chi, then, is movement based on the principles of yin and yang and born out of the Great Void.

Tai chi can also be interpreted as "central pole" or "pillar," like the ridgepole of a house around which all the other parts of the house are arranged and upon which they all depend.

TAI CHI CH'UAN

In one sense, the term t'ai chi is a diminutive, a Western abbreviation of the Chinese term *tai chi ch'uan (taijiquan)*, the full name of the Chinese fighting art. "Ch'uan" means "fist," and the term translated fully means "fighting art based on the laws of the universe."

aphorisms and passages relating to personal conduct and government is traditionally said to be the work of Lao Tzu, a contemporary of the sage Confucius who died in 479 B.C.E. But modern scholarship has established that the *Tao Te Ching* is an anthology of writings by different authors produced around 300 B.C.E., and they refer to it as the *Lao Tzu*. Writings of that era attributed to Chuang Tzu, a second great Taoist thinker, are also known to be a collection of sayings by a number of different people.

Rather than argue over propositions, like the Western philosophers, the philosophers of ancient China sought to make suggestions that might generate ideas and unanswered questions in the mind. A well-known Taoist saying states that as soon as you think

Thirty spokes come together at one hub; because of the empty spaces we have use of a carriage wheel. Mold the clay; because of the empty space we have use of a pot. Cut out doors and windows; because of the empty spaces we have the use of a room.
Thus we gain something by making use of no-thing.

LAO TZU

you know something, a door closes. The Taoist sages sought to remain ever-open to the possibility of learning. Rather than be bound by the limitations of linear thinking, they tried to remain eternally aware of all possible influences on their thinking. For this reason, Taoist writings are full of paradoxes and contradictions intended to challenge limited and inhibiting views on life, and to open the perceptions.

There are many examples of Taoist thought in tai chi. "Plants when they enter life are soft and tender," says the *Lao Tzu*. "When they die they are dry and stiff. Therefore the hard and strong are companions of death. The soft and weak are the companions of life." In tai chi, learning the qualities of softness and understanding its power are essential parts of practice.

Warring states

CHAO	CH'U
CHOU	CHIN
CH'I	YEN
	WEI

• • • • • • • • • •
Area of China c.350 BCE

The *Lao Tzu* was written in China around the 400s BCE, in the midst of the Warring States Period, when numerous small states fought for domination.

CHANGE AND HARMONY

Chinese philosophy is based on a belief in two opposing but complementary forces, yin and yang. Traditionally, yin has been presented as the feminine force, passive, nurturing and soft, and yang as the harder, more active masculine principle. Yin and yang are also the forces of harmony and change, and together they form a balanced whole. When they are not in perfect equilibrium, disorder and disease are said to follow. The interrelationship between change and harmony is the guiding principle behind tai chi, which seeks to establish a dynamic equilibrium between the two.

The process of change may be so gradual as to be barely perceptible, yet it is unceasing and dynamic. The human mind gains profundity and wisdom as the body grows older.

An important theme in tai chi thought is the interplay between yin and yang. Change is a constant in our lives. Nothing is fixed, however solid or permanent it may seem. The Earth moves unceasingly around its orbit, causing the seasons to change and recreating the cycle of birth, life, and death. From the moment of conception to the time of death the body changes ceaselessly. The blood circulates, air is breathed in and out, mind and body mature and age. Throughout our lives we experience not one moment of absolute stillness. Change brings about rhythm, however – every in-breath is followed by an out-breath – and so harmony is maintained.

This ceaseless interplay between change and harmony is perfectly expressed in the yin-yang symbol illustrated opposite. As any condition reaches its fullest point, it already contains the seed of its opposite: in the dark portion is a seed of white; and in the white portion is a seed of black.

The classics say that tai chi moves like a great river. A river is always moving, changing continuously and never the same for a moment, yet it has its own balance and harmony. In tai chi the interplay between yin and yang, the forces of change and harmony, reveals itself in the changing postures and the quality of the movements. Body weight shifts from one leg to the other, awareness moves from inside to out, empty changes to full, open to closed. As each of these movements reaches its conclusion however, the birth of its opposite is already beginning.

It is said that the concepts of yin and yang arose as terms to describe the different sides of a mountain. Yin was the colder, darker, north-facing side and yang the warmer, brighter south side. Gradually the concept was extended: in summer yang force is said to rise and yin force to decline; in autumn yang begins to wane and yin to wax. Life is filled with countless forces and arrangements of opposites: day and night; sound and silence; giving and receiving; fear and courage; sadness and happiness. Taoism teaches that the concepts of yin and yang offer a view of the way things work according to a natural law of change and harmony.

Everyone practicing tai chi is enjoined to embody natural law in their movements in accordance with the constantly changing balance between yin and yang. It may take time and practice, care and concentration, and self-love, but the reward is true harmony of body and mind, the achievement of central equilibrium – which is the essence of tai chi.

YIN-YANG QUALITIES

Below is a list of a few of the many yin and yang qualities. It is important, however, not to see any of them as always being a yin or a yang quality, but as generally belonging to either category under certain circumstances. For example, the Earth receives the seed, protects it, and nurtures it, and so is usually categorized as yin, but if you fall and hit the ground you experience it as hard – as yang.

YIN	YANG
Inward	Outward
Smooth	Rough
Holding	Sending
Receiving	Giving
Listening	Speaking
Dark	Light
Earth	Sky
Soft	Hard
No boundaries	Clear boundaries

THE I CHING

The hexagram Chen from a copy of the I Ching printed in China in the tenth century BCE.

The *I Ching* or *Book of Changes* is one of the five classics of Chinese philosophy and the classic of Taoist thought (see pages 16–17). It is a book of divination and wisdom whose origins are lost in history, although its oldest parts stem from oracles written more than 4,000 years ago. Parts of it have been attributed to a legendary Chinese sage, Fu Hsi, said to have lived 5,000 years ago, but the *Book of Changes* has had many authors as it has itself changed over the ages. It contains elements of Chinese mythology, history, and poetry, and commentaries on its hexagrams including a substantial body said to be the work of Confucius.

The "I" in the title translates both as "change" and as "changelessness." The name is written using characters derived from the ancient Chinese symbols for the sun and the moon. They represent the change from day to night, and its polarity, for the eternal change of day into night into day may also be seen as an unchanging state of equilibrium.

The *I Ching* is a collection of commentaries on 64 hexagrams. These are six-line figures incorporating two trigrams (3-line figures). The lines are unbroken (—) or broken (– –). Originally, an intuitive text explained the meaning of each hexagram and its combination of lines in foretelling the future, but

The philosopher Confucius is said to have written commentaries on the hexagrams.

later texts commented on aspects of the hexagrams' philosophy, interpreting the unbroken lines as yang and the broken lines as yin and offering advice on dealing with life situations.

The book was traditionally consulted using 49 stalks of yarrow, a grass, but it is now usual to throw coins, attributing an unbroken line to one side of the coin and a broken line to the other. The composition of the hexagram depends on the outcome of six throws. You ask the book a question on any subject, and its answer appears in the hexagram you drew with the coins. The text interprets life conditions and situations in terms of yin and yang. Many people find the *I Ching* assists in their decisions by putting them in touch with the part of themselves that makes wise choices.

The relationships between yin and yang give rise to the ba gua or eight diagrams used in the I Ching. Each of the eight basic moves in tai chi corresponds to one of the eight trigrams of the ba gua diagram. They represent the eight conditions of life working in harmony with the tai chi.

THE CHANGES

The *I Ching* explains that the concept of continuous change is the rule:

The Changes is a book
From which one may not hold aloof.
Its tao is forever changing –
Alteration, movement without rest,
Flowing through the six empty places;
Rising and sinking without fixed law,
Firm and yielding transform each other.
They cannot be confined within a rule;
It is only change that is at work here.

The *I Ching* or *Book of Changes*
Richard Wilhelm translation
rendered into English by Cary F. Baynes

太 19 極

THE BIRTH OF TAI CHI

One tradition says that tai chi originated some 5,000 years ago during the reign of China's mythical first emperor, Fu Hsi. Exercises for health are described in a collection of classic writings attributed to one of his successors, the legendary Yellow Emperor, Huang Ti, who is said to have founded the traditional Chinese system of medicine. The principles of the art were established by Taoist recluses who retired from the world to live as hermits, immersing themselves in a study of nature. And it evolved during turbulent periods in China's history as a martial art called t'ai chi ch'uan.

Although tai chi is thought to have originated before the first millennium, the earliest known references date from the T'ang Dynasty (ACE 618–960). They describe "patterns' of tai chi practiced by recluses who had retired to China's mountain regions to study nature (see pages 16–17). These "patterns" are believed to have been chains of movements which were perhaps the precursor of the tai chi form.

The early tai chi teachers remain semi-mythical figures. Chang San-feng is an exception, a colorful figure, larger than life, and said to have been more than 6 feet tall and a powerful fighter. No one knows whether he really existed or when. Some sources say he lived during the 900s, while the official history of the Ming Dynasty claims he was born in 1247. Nevertheless, he is credited as the founder of a spiritual fighting art called Wudang kung fu.

The Ming Dynasty history records that Chang Sang-feng studied under a Taoist recluse living in the mountains of northwest China, then studied martial arts at the Shaolin Temple Monastery near Zhengzhou in modern Henan. The Shaolin Temple is famous as the crucible of the martial systems now practiced worldwide. Shaolin Temple boxing or kung fu is a hard martial art, a system based on pitting force against force.

However, it is said that in tai chi a process leads the player from body to mind to spirit, and eventually back to the Great Void to merge with the cosmos. Chang San-feng apparently followed this path, which led him to further studies at the Purple Summit Temple on the Wudang Shan, a mountain held sacred by Taoists since from time immemorial they

Training at the Shaolin Temple, birthplace of the Chinese martial arts.

had retired there to seek the Tao (see pages 16–17). Chang San-feng spent nine years there, it is said, studying nature, and was struck by the martial potential of yielding while watching a fight between a snake and a bird (see page 152). He modified his kung fu style, replacing training methods such as lifting weights and hitting sandbags with mind-focusing techniques like visualization, and the cultivation of energy through qigung (see page 156). From this point, China's "soft" or "internal" fighting arts: ba gua, hsingi, and t'ai chi ch'uan may have developed.

As the peaceful and prosperous Ming Dynasty declined in the 1600s, to be replaced by conquerors from Manchuria, hand-to-hand battlefield combat was a frequent reality and personal combat skills were at a premium among the imperial forces. New martial styles evolved during this era, and the internal or soft styles were established. Foremost among these was the Chen style of tai chi, founded by Chen Wang-t'ing, a soldier in the imperial Ming armies who served under a respected general, Ch'i Chi-guang. Ch'i wrote the *Classic of kung fu*, setting out the principles of what became Chen style. However, it is also claimed that Chen studied under the author of the now-classic *Treatise on T'ai Chi Ch'uan*, Wang Tsung-yueh, whose lineage could be traced back to the legendary fighter Chang San-feng. It was Chen who first spoke of t'ai chi ch'uan rather than Wudang kung fu.

Three founding fathers of Taoism, the ancient Chinese philosophy on which Tai Chi is based.

THE ORIGINS OF T'AI CHI CH'UAN

Little is known of the earliest tai chi exercises or patterns. The first recorded reference to t'ai chi ch'uan occurs in the classic text, *The Method of Attaining Enlightenment through Observing the Scripture*, written by Cheng Ling-hsi who in the early 900s is said to have practiced The 14 Patterns of Tai Chi Training. By the early 1800s the first recognized tai chi style is known from Chen family records to have emerged in the clan's villages in Henan Province.

T'ang Dynasty (C.E. 618–906)
A Taoist priest, Li Tao-tsu, at a monastery on the sacred Wudang Shan, practices Primordial Longfist, similar to The 37 Patterns.

Liang Dynasty (C.E. 907–923)
Cheng Ling-hsi, a Taoist, practiced The 14 Patterns of Tai Chi, founded by another recluse, Hao Gong-yueh.

Ming Dynasty (1368–1644) Early 1600s
General Ch'i Chi-guang writes the *Classic of Kung fu*, setting out principles on which Chen-style tai chi is based.

T'ang Dynasty (C.E. 618–906)
Hsu Hsun-ping, a hermit, practiced the 37 Patterns of tai chi, also called Changjian (Yangtse) Longfist after the name of China's longest river, because of its ceaseless flow.

Ming Dynasty Mid-1600s
Chen Wang-t'ing (1600–1680), a soldier, develops a new Wudang kung fu style, calling it t'ai chi ch'uan.

Ch'ing Dynasty Early 1800s
Chen You-ben develops a new Chen form, while his relative, Chen Chang-hsing, continues teaching Chen-style Old Form.

太 21 極

An elderly man practices a tai chi form beside Green Lake in Kunming Province, China.

By the 1800s tai chi was at its zenith as a fighting art, and the Chen style was well established. However, it was still taught only to members of the Chen family (see pages 20–21).

In the early 1800s a student from a poor family, Yang Lu-ch'an, found work in the household of the clan head, Chen Chang-xing. It is recounted that Yang spied on tai chi sessions, learning by observation. One day he surprised the family by offering to fight a stranger who had challenged Chen Chang-xing. Yang fought so well in authentic Chen style, beating the stranger, that it was obvious that he had been secretly learning the style. Magnanimously, Chen accepted his apologies and accepted Yang as a student.

Yang Lu-ch'an traveled China as a Chen family representative, offering challenges to fighters, and because he always beat his opponents he was nicknamed "Ever-Victorious." He is said to have been appointed to teach Chen-style t'ai chi ch'uan to the household of the Ch'ing Emperor. Chen style is dynamic and physically demanding with postures that clearly demonstrate a polarity of fast and slow, small and large movements. To adapt the style for courtiers who had not trained from early youth – or perhaps to preserve the Chen family style – Yang omitted the more vigorous and strenuous movements, creating a gentler form of tai chi.

Today, while Chen is recognized as the oldest of the three principal tai chi styles practiced today, a shorter version of Yang's style is most widely taught.

The third style was developed by Yang's student, Wu Yu-hsiang, who also studied with the Chen family, so his style incorporates features of both. These three styles have given rise to numerous derivatives. For example, in the later 1800s Wu Ch'uan-yu developed a second Wu style, called the Small Style and characterized by a forward lean. The two Wu styles

are written with different Chinese characters but sound the same, so both are written as "Wu" in the Roman alphabet. It is worth knowing which lineage is taught before studying Wu style.

Sun Lu-t'ang, a master of the arts of ba gua and hsingi, was 50 when he began learning a derivative of the first Wu style, which had been modified by Wu Yu-hsiang's students and was taught as the Hou or Li style. Sun developed his own version, characterized by small circular movements and high stances.

While China's imperial governments generally discouraged the fighting arts, the Communist government under Mao Zedong treasured the people's tai chi heritage. In 1949 they set up the Wushu Council ("wushu" means "art of powerful movement") to formulate a style that would improve people's health, and to structure tai chi as a competitive sport. A new style called the Beijing 24 Step Form was the result, created by Master Li Tienzhi, who condensed the essential elements of Yang Style. A 48-step standard competition form was also developed from elements of the Yang, Wu, Chen and Hou styles. Beijing style is now taught worldwide.

One outstanding teacher who bridges the classic tai chi styles with 20th-century developments is Cheng Man-ch'ing. A doctor of Chinese herbal medicine, he studied under Yang Cheng-fu, grandson of the famous founder of the Yang style. A fine fighter, Yang eliminated foot-stamping, straight-punching, and jumping from his grandfather's form and made the movements bigger, smoother, and rounder, developing the now-classic Yang-style Big Form of 108 postures. In the 1930s Cheng Man-ch'ing simplified Yang Cheng-fu's form, reducing it to 37 postures. His Short Form retains the elements of Yang's style, but is easier to learn. In the 1960s Cheng, now widely known and respected, opened a tai chi school in New York. Today, his style is popular worldwide.

TAI CHI SPREADS WORLDWIDE

During the 1800s t'ai chi ch'uan flourished and the classic schools were established. New warfare technology diminished tai chi's role as a battlefield art so that the tai chi families no longer needed to keep their arts secret. Since 1900 tai chi has become accessible to ordinary Chinese people, and has spread beyond the frontiers of China out into Asia and westward, to North America, Britain, Australia and New Zealand, and into Europe.

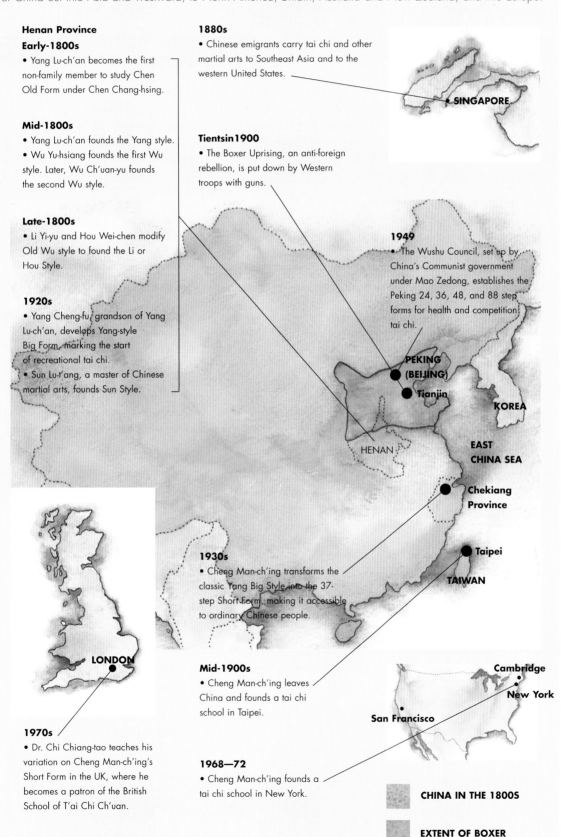

Henan Province
Early-1800s
• Yang Lu-ch'an becomes the first non-family member to study Chen Old Form under Chen Chang-hsing.

Mid-1800s
• Yang Lu-ch'an founds the Yang style.
• Wu Yu-hsiang founds the first Wu style. Later, Wu Ch'uan-yu founds the second Wu style.

Late-1800s
• Li Yi-yu and Hou Wei-chen modify Old Wu style to found the Li or Hou Style.

1920s
• Yang Cheng-fu, grandson of Yang Lu-ch'an, develops Yang-style Big Form, marking the start of recreational tai chi.
• Sun Lu-t'ang, a master of Chinese martial arts, founds Sun Style.

1880s
• Chinese emigrants carry tai chi and other martial arts to Southeast Asia and to the western United States.

SINGAPORE

Tientsin 1900
• The Boxer Uprising, an anti-foreign rebellion, is put down by Western troops with guns.

1949
• The Wushu Council, set up by China's Communist government under Mao Zedong, establishes the Peking 24, 36, 48, and 88 step forms for health and competition tai chi.

PEKING (BEIJING)
Tianjin
KOREA
HENAN
EAST CHINA SEA
Chekiang Province
Taipei
TAIWAN

LONDON

1930s
• Cheng Man-ch'ing transforms the classic Yang Big Style into the 37-step Short Form, making it accessible to ordinary Chinese people.

Mid-1900s
• Cheng Man-ch'ing leaves China and founds a tai chi school in Taipei.

Cambridge
New York
San Francisco

1970s
• Dr. Chi Chiang-tao teaches his variation on Cheng Man-ch'ing's Short Form in the UK, where he becomes a patron of the British School of T'ai Chi Ch'uan.

1968—72
• Cheng Man-ch'ing founds a tai chi school in New York.

CHINA IN THE 1800S

EXTENT OF BOXER UPRISING

A HEALING ART

Tai chi is best known in the West as a system of exercises to benefit health, prevent degenerative illnesses, and promote longevity. It stimulates circulation, aligns misplaced bones, mobilizes the joints, stimulates and maintains vital organs, and improves balance and coordination. It improves the breathing, which revitalizes body and brain. But tai chi is a holistic practice and it also trains the mind to focus and concentrate. It widens sensitivity and the capacity to feel, so that people who practice become more awake, alive, and responsive.

The following chapters show many different ways in which tai chi can benefit health of body and mind. The bow and arrow stance, for instance, makes the ankles more flexible, while Single Whip opens the lungs and improves the breathing. Through exercise, tai chi works with the body to support and encourage its natural capacity for healing. It does this by building energy. Practicing the techniques correctly raises chi, or life energy, which strengthens the immune system and improves health, and jin or whole body energy, also called intrinsic energy, which improves coordination.

Tai chi movements build energy, beginning at a low level and, with the right kind of fuel, growing into a steady, strong blaze. This cannot be hurried or forced but must be carefully watched and fed. Tai chi movements generate warmth, which is often accompanied by a sense of fullness. After perhaps half an hour of practice the body may feel as if it is humming. After a training session this can be felt as heat energy in certain parts of the body. It can be detected in the hands, for example, by pressing the palms together lightly – they seem to radiate heat.

When tai chi is practiced regularly, a combination of mindset, visualization, body shape (the positions made by the body), and movement create the conditions for streams of energy to flow vigorously through the body, stimulating the internal systems. It is said in the ancient writings on tai chi that the chi (life energy) follows the mind. This means that each posture cultivates a different kind of energy flow, depending on visualization and the body shapes it makes. The hands are transmitters for this energy, and as the mind's intention changes from receiving to giving and inward to outward, the hands become charged as a result of the passage of large amounts of information through them.

Healing is a natural force and the body wants to heal itself. This perspective makes it logical to stand aside to allow healing to occur, rather than trying to make it happen. Healing can only be encouraged, it cannot be made to take place, any more than a plant can be made to grow. The role of the individual in the process is to try, through tai chi, to create the conditions in which energy can flow, and to give the body time to heal itself.

SELF-HEALING

Tai chi is a healing art and just practicing it generates the energy that makes healing possible. The following exercises act as a useful complement to this aspect of tai chi. They can be done at any time, but they are especially effective immediately after practice.

2 *Release your hands, place your right hand on the lower tantien and your left hand on the center of your chest. Again, hold this position for two to five minutes, concentrating on gathering into yourself and charging your batteries.*

HANDS ON

1 *Place your left hand on the lower tantien energy center, just below the navel, and your right hand on top of it. Rest in this position for two to five minutes. Concentrate on gathering into yourself and charging your batteries.*

The feet work hard, yet they tend to be neglected. They benefit from massage, especially before and after practice.

MASSAGE

The idea in massage for tai chi is to develop your spontaneity and intuition for self-healing. There are no special strokes to apply, and you need not worry about direction or pressure of stroke. Begin by following your own feelings about what to do. Rub briskly if you want to, or stroke gently.

MASSAGING THE FACE

Bring both hands to your chin and slowly draw them up over your face, back through your hair, and down your neck. Repeat five times.

MASSAGING THE EARS

Rub the lobes of each ear vigorously, then run your finger and thumb around the rim of the ear and back again to each ear lobe.

MASSAGING THE EYES

Close your eyes and (always with clean hands) stroke the upper eyelids lightly with the middle finger from close to the top of the nose out to the side of the head. Repeat this action at least seven times, then stroke the bottom eyelid in the same way.

MASSAGING THE FEET

Massaging your feet stimulates the nerve-endings and is relaxing and comforting. Hold or rub your feet one at a time for at least two minutes each.

MASSAGING THE HANDS

Massage stimulates the many nerve-endings in the hands, improving the circulation and bringing life to them. Gently or vigorously rub your hands. Pay attention to each finger and both thumbs, the palms and the backs of the hands.

HEALING OTHERS

Massage for tai chi can be reassuring, so offering to massage relatives or friends is a way of helping them through touch. Explore for yourself and discover how the healing energy generated in tai chi practice can help you, your friends and family.

FOOT-HOLDING AND INTUITIVE FOOT MASSAGE

The simple technique of foot-holding embodies the principle of "not doing" perfectly. For the best effect the person to be massaged should lie down comfortably, or, if this is not possible, sit in a chair with the knees and legs supported on a stool or cushions. Rest your hands on the other person's ankles or feet and do nothing for at least 10 minutes. Notice how energy builds in both bodies. This demonstrates the two-way nature of healing and the positive feedback that begins with tai chi practice. Intuitive foot massage is stimulating and comforting. Simply massage the other person's feet in any way that occurs to you.

DISPELLING A HEADACHE

Ask your friend to sit comfortably. Rest your right hand on his or her forehead and your left hand on the back of the neck, and keep your hands still for at least 3 minutes. Now move your hands about 9 inches away from your friend's head and neck, imagining them offering a healing space into which the "dis-ease" of the headache can melt. Finish by placing both of your hands in light contact for about a minute.

A few minutes of gentle massage can release tension and remove the pain of a headache.

SEVEN QUALITIES

Every posture in tai chi is a combination of seven basic qualities. Central to these qualities is the concept of yin and yang, the forces of change and harmony, one of the fundamental principles of Chinese philosophy. Like yin and yang, the basic qualities of tai chi are almost all polarities: open and closed; full and empty. The exception is the seventh, central equilibrium. Consciousness of these seven qualities pervades every aspect of a posture while it is being performed. They are the focus of the mind, they are expressed in the movements, and they are the message communicated through the very spirit of the posture.

The concepts of yin and yang underlie every movement in tai chi. The form (see page 14) is a sequence of postures in a state of perpetual transformation, a cycle of harmony and change. A posture begins, grows, reaches a fullness, and starts to empty. Its emptying is the growth of the next one.

To fulfil their task of restoring perfect equilibrium between yin and yang, the movements of the form must be executed with the correct technique and mind intent (mindset or attitude). But for a beginner, body and mind are too fully occupied with learning the sequence of movements and the technique – exactly where a foot or a hand should be at each moment in a posture – to experience the qualities of each movement. So before beginning the form, devote time to learning about movement, focusing on moving in certain ways and experiencing the qualities in movement.

The postures move between the polarities of open and closed. At every moment, every part of the body is open or closed, so studying one's own posture and trying to see where it is open and where closed gives an idea of what these concepts mean. The arms and shoulders are usually a good way of telling. Squeezing the upper arms tightly against the ribs will show how closed feels, and lifting the arms outward as when welcoming a friend is an open gesture. This exercise is echoed in the Lifting Hands posture (see page 96). The arms are open at the start, and then they begin to close.

Balance improves by standing on each leg in turn for a few minutes each day. This strengthens the legs and improves the coordination, but it also makes you feel different. Physical equilibrium infiltrates the mental and emotional spheres of your being.

The polarities of full and empty give the body mobility. To take a step forward, people tend to drop their weight onto the leg being moved, but in tai chi balance is held in one leg, leaving the other free to move. The weight empties from one leg and fills the other, as the exercise opposite seeks to demonstrate, increasing mobility. Emptying is vividly demonstrated in Pushing Hands (see pages 148–51). The person receiving a push does not so much retreat as create an empty space for the partner's push to fall into. Full is best demonstrated in Standing Like A Mountain on page 39, a stance which gives solid resistance to a push.

Full or empty, open or closed, the body must be in balance.

Without equilibrium a posture will lose its structure, becoming too open or too closed. Structure lends strength to a posture. Central equilibrium is the foundation of every stance and the hub of every movement, the thread that runs through tai chi. When a posture is based on central equilibrium, the body is aligned between earth and sky, so it is perfectly balanced, and it retains these qualities of alignment and central equilibrium however small or large a movement it makes.

Beginners unfamiliar with having to relate qualities such as empty or closed to movements of the body find it hard to combine the mental concept with the physical experience. Familiarity makes these qualities more and more interesting, however, since they affect almost every aspect of every tai chi movement. Practicing them therefore needs to become part of regular practice.

YIN AND YANG

Create your own body shapes to express qualities of yin and yang described on pages 18–19. As a guide for yin, use soft, round, smooth, flowing shapes to embody the qualities. For yang use hard, angular, and linear as your guiding concepts. Play with all these possibilities and add your own.

Yin body shape

Yang body shape

OPEN AND CLOSED

Here you can discover how open and closed feel when expressed as movement. As you practice, the polarity intensifies the experience of the movement.

1 *Stand with your feet apart, lift your arms up and out in a welcoming gesture, and imagine each body part and your feelings opening up.*

2 *Slowly draw your arms in, crossing them over your chest, contemplating this closed position. End by lowering your arms and standing erect for a while.*

FULL AND EMPTY

The second exercise expands the first to make greater demands on your imagination. Imagine yourself as an empty vessel; picture the reality of fullness.

1 *Standing with your feet apart, transfer your weight from leg to leg, back and forth, then slow down to slow motion for about four minutes. Notice how you feel as one leg fills and the other empties.*

2 *Imagine colored liquid filling you from your feet up. Experience every cell in your body expanding as it rises, moving your arms out as if you are inflating. Then close your eyes and imagine your body is hollow. Visualize yourself becoming emptiness.*

SEVEN STEPS TO PROGRESS

Tai chi offers more than exercises for health, it also provides a program for self-development. The influential teachers Cheng Man-ch'ing and Chi Chiang-tao mapped out a sevenfold path to tai chi practice. For just as the postures are composed of seven basic qualities, so there are seven dimensions to practice, seven steps to progress through the form.

Imagine trying to stop the flow of a river. Imagine trying to make it flow faster. The way of tai chi is always to flow with the river. Beginners may be surprised to find how effectively they have been conditioned to fight the river's natural flow, or to try to dominate it. This is to use force against force. We are conditioned into this way of thinking as we are trained to keep to timetables and meet deadlines rather than follow the natural rhythms of our body and mind.

Tai chi teaches people to correct this imbalance by becoming alert to intelligence from within while learning to listen to what is happening outside and to respond to others. It teaches patience, the ability to wait, alert but quiet, for the right moment to move or act, rather than fill gaps between activity with impatient non-action.

By exercising the body, tai chi raises energy and enhances 'the mind's abilities and the spirit's potential. When tai chi movements are performed correctly, they work to calm and focus the mind, so that mind, energy, and body work in harmony. The spirit is released, inspiration and creative energies have the freedom to develop, and space is created for essential, natural, human qualities to emerge.

Tai chi teaches you to respond to a partner's movements. Sumo wrestlers use force against force.

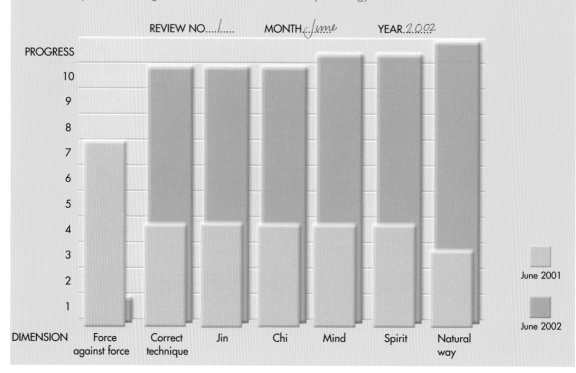

MAPPING TAI CHI PRACTICE

The seven dimensions of tai chi practice, described on the page opposite, may be represented by a graph on which you map your progress along the path to natural way. The vertical axis measures your progress on a scale from 1 to 10. A teacher might help you assess your abilities in each area. Draw a new graph to review progress after a year. Your tendency to use force against force should have fallen and your energy and coordination have risen.

REVIEW NO....1.... MONTH June YEAR 2002

PROGRESS

June 2001
June 2002

DIMENSION Force against force Correct technique Jin Chi Mind Spirit Natural way

FORCE AGAINST FORCE

Have you been trying to dominate by blocking your partner's responses, or responding too quickly, before your partner stops pushing? If so, you are using force against force, so mark a high score on the graph. In this interaction you enter into a dialogue, inviting your partner to respond to your push. Do not try to force one. When receiving a push, listen as the movement unfolds, knowing that each push has its lifetime. Do not stop it by force, but move in response to the other person. This is the natural way.

CORRECT TECHNIQUE

Perfecting tai chi technique is hard work. It seems impossible to get all parts of the body in exactly the right place and position while they are moving or preparing to move. However, although the rules of tai chi are challenging, they are effective. Hands and feet need to be correctly aligned, placed, and arranged because it enables you to reap the richest reward from practice. And bear in mind that improvement often comes without a struggle. Working on the mind, for instance, sharpens concentration, which brings about improvements in technique.

JIN OR WHOLE BODY ENERGY

Beginners feel all left feet, and every part of the body seems to go its own way. As practice evolves, feet, legs and pelvis, spine, arms and hands feel more connected, and as expertise develops, movements of head and body begin to feel coordinated. There comes a time when breathing and movement of all parts of the body follow one rhythm, and this cohesion is jin, or whole body energy. With time and practice your body can become solid, or, depending on the type of jin you need, light, like air.

CHI OR LIFE FORCE ENERGY

Tai chi movements stimulate the chi circulating in the body and the musculoskeletal system and they exercise the internal organs, and open the meridians (see page 54). This, combined with the rhythm of tai chi movements, allows chi to build. Chi is said to be led by the mind, so resting the mind quietly in the lower tantien energy center (see page 57) after practice also builds chi. People often feel contentment and greater vitality after practice.

MIND

Cultivating awareness is the key to mind control – if your mind keeps returning to one of the day's events while you are practicing, acknowledge it: "I'm thinking about this person's remark as I step forward." Notice where your mind is directed as you move back, and again as you lift your arm. This approach dissolves the tension, creates space, and calms the mind. Soon, there will be moments when it becomes absorbed in working out a tricky move, and the moments will extend to minutes. Then you find your mind making visualizations at will.

SPIRIT

There is a dynamic equilibrium between earth and spirit in tai chi. The way to spirit is through the earthing of the body, and the stronger the connection with the earth, the greater the possibilities for spirit. One of the joys of practice is allowing the body to radiate the spirit that powers each posture – the spirit of fire or of clarity. Bring the spirit of the moment spontaneously into practice. You may feel poised, spirit bursting, like a cat about to pounce, then you might become quiet, nurturing the spirit inside.

NATURAL WAY

The goal of self-development through tai chi is to follow the natural way, so emerging into the seventh dimension is a confirmation of progress. It comes about through letting go of the binding patterns of force against force, becoming receptive to the natural way of things, and learning to wait for the right moment to move. Striving to achieve natural way is to use force against force. Attaining natural way is a sevenfold process. The qualities work together to realign the whole person toward natural way.

MIND GAME

This visualization may take a while to become real, but it will show how your mind and your energy can work together.

Turn your left palm toward you. Point the fingers of your right hand toward your left palm keeping them about six inches away. Imagine the fingers of your right hand are brushes. Paint strokes very slowly over your left hand. At first you may not sense anything, but soon you will feel the light brush strokes moving across the sensitive palm of your hand as clearly as if you were really painting it.

2

A BODY-BASED
PRACTICE

MOVEMENT, HEALTH, AND BODY AWARENESS

The body is an extraordinary, wonderful instrument. It is mechanically well designed and physically intricate, yet it also houses the spirit. The body bestows on its owner the gift of movement, yet people living a modern lifestyle rarely if ever make the most of this ability, and many have forgotten or never discovered how fast, how slowly, or how far the body and its constituent parts are capable of moving. Yet not only is the body designed to move, it needs to, in order to stay healthy. Tai chi provides a form of exercise that offers a remedy for the ills of modern living, a supportive answer to the body's need to move.

A sedentary lifestyle now can mean mobility problems later on in life.

While they are still developing in their mother's womb, unborn infants know how to move. They swim, dance, push, wriggle, and kick. Immediately after birth, babies move instinctively and without inhibition, and during the early years, movement plays an essential part in childhood learning and personal development. Young children crawl, roll, totter, and fall; as they grow they play on swings, slides, roundabouts, and with each other. A child's world is to a large extent body-based.

Relatively few adults in modern industrial countries still have to cut hay, harvest crops, fetch water, or chop wood by hand in order to survive. Most are relieved of such tiresome tasks and chores by modern economic organization, which uses machines to perform repetitive jobs, releasing people to attend to tasks carried out by telephone, pager, fax, or computer, reached by automobile, rail or air link, e-mail or internet. People are rarely forced by their work to stretch or stress their bodies.

Problems tend to begin shortly after the point where demands cease to be made of the body. Arthritis, for example, is associated not with overstressing the joints, but with underexercising them. One physiologist has estimated that 150 years of good service could normally be expected from the superbly designed joints of the human frame. Yet they waste away, working at a fraction of their potential, while the body sits unmoving on office chairs and at boardroom tables, or lounges supine on sofas.

By placing emphasis on mental achievement and a globalizing electronic culture, contemporary living draws energy from the body into the head, simply because exercising the mind draws blood to the brain. The ratio of mental and emotional stimulation to physical activity was reversed during the 20th century, and for many the reversal took place in fewer than 50 years. Modern work stresses the mind but fails to work the body, making true rest difficult to achieve.

Society today is predominantly sedentary. Anyone doing an office or a driving job is required to sit for long periods. Then, at the end of the day they rest in a sitting position, unlike most animals, which tend to rest lying down. Tribal peoples who retain their ancient customs often rest by squatting, kneeling, or lying. Modern people sit on a chair, on the tail of the spine, a position which far from being restful is a kind of slump. In time, this bad posture can result in a tendency to asthma, lower back trouble, and prolapsed (displaced) internal organs.

Sitting back to relax – or, more accurately, to collapse and watch TV, sets up another dynamic.

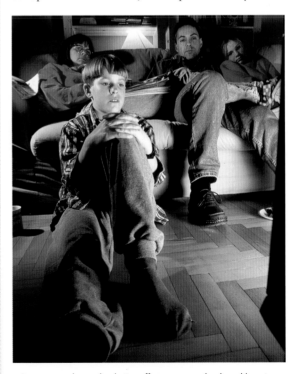

Poor posture has a deadening effect on energy levels and learning ability, creativity, outlook, and mood.

The body responds generously to the visual stimuli presented on a screen, by producing an emotional response in the form of energy which needs to find expression. Cheering when a favored team scores and grumbling when it fails release only some of this energy. Physical activity redresses the balance, so one might react to the excitement of a goal by standing up or hit the furniture when distressed by a referee's decision. Aware of the need for an outlet for such unexpressed energy, people tend to follow logic and take up some form of exercise. It is all too easy, however, to overreact and pummel the body with exercise. Activity that is too vigorous can shock the body and injure its systems.

Tai chi is quality movement. It is physically demanding, yet it works with the body to encourage the gradual developing of strength and reviving of natural openness and coordination. This process is not something that can be hurried, however. Tai chi is an art that needs to be mastered through gradual learning and practice, but the benefits of investing time and effort in it become apparent very early on.

Like a door, the body must be kept moving to prevent its hinge joints – and other types of joint – from seizing up, and tai chi works to condition the elements of the human frame. It promotes greater understanding of the body's natural alignment and stance, encouraging the habit of good posture. Its movements continually turn the spine, an action that gradually repositions misplaced organs, stimulating them at the same time through an internal form of massage. The tai chi movements dissipate excess nervous tension held in the body and so help balance the nervous system.

Working out can demand too much of the body without considering its needs and tolerances.

Through apparently simple exercises, such as standing on one leg, tai chi stimulates the muscle groups to work together. In this way, balance plays a part all through practice in toning up the musculoskeletal system. Continued through life it prevents the joints of the hips and limbs from degenerating.

We are fortunate as humans to have exceptional bodies. Our unique upright stance gives us a greater potential for movements than creatures who walk on four legs. By comparison with a sea creature, such as a dolphin, the physical capabilities of humans seem inferior when in water, yet it is the human who can walk out of the water onto the land, play volleyball, climb a tree, paint a picture, and cook a meal. Each day, our bodies perform wonders for us.

But do we know our bodies? Learning tai chi helps raise body awareness. The next few pages present some of the workings of the body from a holistic point of view, from the mechanical structure of the frame to the internal systems and the location of the energy centers, and it shows how tai chi encourages the development of a personal connection with the body.

Tai chi is a holistic practice, its movements exercise the whole body, not just individual muscles or muscle groups. It works gently to encourage the body's natural harmony.

THE SKELETON

The body's architecture provides the framework for the extraordinary variety of movement and bodily expression that is tai chi. The art makes full use of the combination of dexterity, flexibility, articulation, and movement capabilities which the skeleton, aided by ligaments, muscles, and tendons, makes possible. It is not essential to learn anatomy before practicing tai chi, but knowing the basics of body architecture will deepen understanding of the tai chi postures. It will also give a sense of wonder at the sheer variety of movements the human body can perform, which is unparalleled in the rest of the animal kingdom.

The skeleton is the body's frame, supporting it and giving it shape. The bony cavities of the skull, the rib cage, and the pelvic girdle provide protection for the body's vital organs – the brain, the lungs, the organs of digestion, and the sexual organs. The appearance of the skeleton is so extraordinary it can be hard to believe that it is us, yet its design has evolved over millions of years to make it perfectly adapted for movement. The girders of a building are bolted into a rigid framework, but the skeletal bones are connected by joints held together by ligaments and operated by muscles. This system gives the body mobility.

Tai chi actively increases mobility in all the joints of the body, maintaining an especially strong focus on the ankles, knees, hips, shoulders, elbows, wrists, and spine. It achieves this mainly by encouraging the joints to open, that is, to relax completely (see page 27).

Although the word "skeleton" means "dried up,"

the bones of the skeleton are far from being dead and desiccated. Bone is living tissue made of active cells served by blood vessels and nerves, and the tissues in its spongy center carry out the vital task of making bone marrow. The red blood cells, which transport oxygen, are formed in the bone marrow along with white blood cells, which fight infection. Bones are therefore fundamental to the body's immune system.

Tai chi attributes another important function to the bone marrow. The teacher Cheng Man-ch'ing (see pages 22–23) described the cultivation of chi in the lower tantien energy center, how it warms the fluids of the body and fills the hollow spaces of the bones. An adhesive substance forms, which turns into marrow and plates the insides of the bones like nickel or gold, giving them greater weight and pure hardness. It is said that the arms of Cheng's master, Yang Cheng-fu, were heavier than average because of this process.

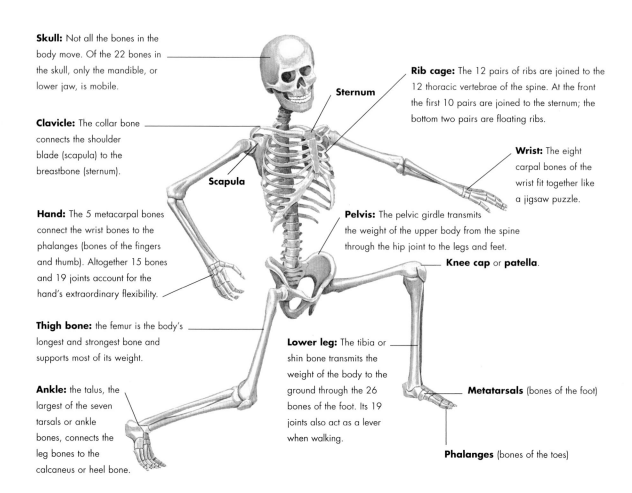

Skull: Not all the bones in the body move. Of the 22 bones in the skull, only the mandible, or lower jaw, is mobile.

Clavicle: The collar bone connects the shoulder blade (scapula) to the breastbone (sternum).

Hand: The 5 metacarpal bones connect the wrist bones to the phalanges (bones of the fingers and thumb). Altogether 15 bones and 19 joints account for the hand's extraordinary flexibility.

Thigh bone: the femur is the body's longest and strongest bone and supports most of its weight.

Ankle: the talus, the largest of the seven tarsals or ankle bones, connects the leg bones to the calcaneus or heel bone.

Sternum

Rib cage: The 12 pairs of ribs are joined to the 12 thoracic vertebrae of the spine. At the front the first 10 pairs are joined to the sternum; the bottom two pairs are floating ribs.

Wrist: The eight carpal bones of the wrist fit together like a jigsaw puzzle.

Scapula

Pelvis: The pelvic girdle transmits the weight of the upper body from the spine through the hip joint to the legs and feet.

Knee cap or **patella.**

Lower leg: The tibia or shin bone transmits the weight of the body to the ground through the 26 bones of the foot. Its 19 joints also act as a lever when walking.

Metatarsals (bones of the foot)

Phalanges (bones of the toes)

THE BONES

All bones begin as flexible cartilage, which forms in the womb. As the baby grows the cartilage is gradually converted into bones, which continue to lengthen and grow until the end of the teen years. A baby's skeleton has more than 350 bones, many of which fuse as the baby grows, so that an adult's skeleton has only 206 bones. Women have the same number as men, but men have broader shoulder bones and a longer rib cage, and their skeleton is usually broader and longer than that of a woman, which has a wider pelvic opening.

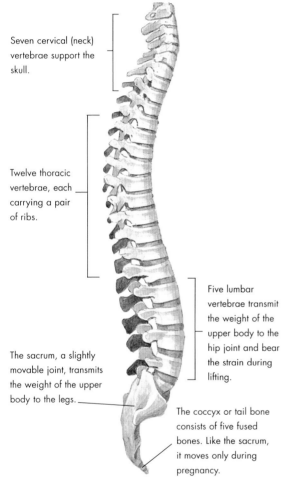

Seven cervical (neck) vertebrae support the skull.

Twelve thoracic vertebrae, each carrying a pair of ribs.

The sacrum, a slightly movable joint, transmits the weight of the upper body to the legs.

Five lumbar vertebrae transmit the weight of the upper body to the hip joint and bear the strain during lifting.

The coccyx or tail bone consists of five fused bones. Like the sacrum, it moves only during pregnancy.

The bones, or vertebrae, and joints of the spine

THE SPINE

The spine is made up of 33 bones but only 25 joints because the last four bones are fused to form the coccyx (tail bone) and the five bones above them are fused to form the sacrum, which wedges into the back of the pelvic girdle. Each bone is called a vertebra, and the vertebrae form groups, each of which differs slightly in its function. The vertebrae are separated by discs of cartilage, forming a slightly movable joint. These cartilaginous joints work together, allowing the spine to move forward, backward, and sideways. The spinal cord, a bundle of major nerve fibers, travels along a channel through the center of the vertebrae from the pelvis to join the brain.

THE SACRUM

The broad shield-shaped bone at the base of the spine transmits the weight of the body from the fifth lumbar vertebra sideways to the pelvic girdle. The sacrum ("sacred bone") forms the bottom bend of the spine's s-curve. It forms a slightly movable joint with the fifth lumbar vertebra, but its side "wings" (called "alas") fit perfectly into the corresponding surfaces of the pelvic girdle, and ligaments secure the sacroiliac joints so firmly as to make them almost immobile. They move only in women during childbirth, when hormones temporarily soften the ligaments. The sacrum plays a fundamental role in the mechanics of tai chi movement and is a key reference point in the interpretation of tai chi presented in this book.

THE JOINTS

Beside the cartilaginous joints in the spine and the synovial joints between the sacrum and the pelvic girdle, the body has many different moving joints. Three principal ones are shown below. Although tai chi movements exercise all the body's joints, they focus on opening and exercising the joints of the ankles, knees, hips, shoulders, elbows, and wrists, and on maintaining the mobility of the multi-jointed spine.

BALL AND SOCKET JOINT
A ball and socket joint is where the rounded head of one bone fits into a socket or hole in the adjoining bone. Ball and socket joints at the shoulders and hip allow the arms and legs almost 360° of movement.

Hip joint

HINGE JOINT
The knee, toes, fingers and elbow are examples of hinge joints, which permit bending and straightening in one direction. A rounded bulge in one bone fits into a corresponding hollow in an adjoining bone. The two bones are held together by ligaments and encased in a capsule filled with a lubricating fluid.

Elbow joint

PIVOT JOINT
The first two cervical vertebrae in the neck form a pivot joint. A protuberance in the second cervical vertebra, called the axis, fits into a ring formed in the vertebra above it, called the atlas. This joint allows the neck to pivot from side to side through more than 180°. The skull rests in a groove on the atlas, or first cervical vertebra, forming a joint which allows the head to nod up and down.

Atlas

Axis

Neck joint

THE MUSCLES

One of the first things people notice when they start tai chi is that their legs begin to feel different. To some it can be a shock to find that the gentle, flowing movements, so attractive to watch, can require such hard work from the muscles of their thighs and calves. But it is the demands made on the muscle groups of the legs combined with the ability to fully relax muscles elsewhere in the body that gives tai chi its unique grace of movement.

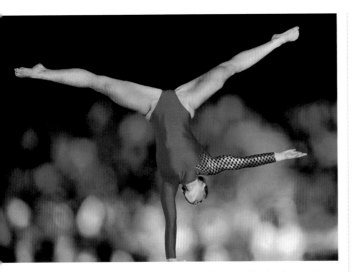

Gymnasts may seem to achieve the impossible, but they are in fact demonstrating the full flexibility that the skeletal muscles can achieve.

During infancy we learn to use the muscles under our conscious control, but we often need to retrain some of them through tai chi, especially those of the lower limbs which play a major role in bodily expression. For this reason, after a tai chi posture is learned there may be a time-gap before it can be performed with real ease. This is the maturing time the muscles need to strengthen and learn the new movements.

The muscles execute commands from the brain carried along the motor nerves. The time-lapse between thinking of moving and carrying out a movement may be scarcely perceptible, and for the muscles to be able to react so quickly, the nervous system maintains them in a half-alert state called muscle tone. This ensures that voluntary movements are not started from cold.

This link with the nervous system means that emotional stress registers in the muscles, however. Feelings of fear or anxiety show as a measurable rise in muscle tone. This reaction is appropriate as a "fight-or-flight" response, enabling the body to react instantly to an emergency, but people who suffer from recurrent fear or anxiety may be held in a permanent state of tension and find it hard to rest and impossible to relax. This is chronic stress (see pages 166–67).

On one level tai chi deals with stress by relaxing the muscles. "Soft" (see page 65) does not mean flaccid, but a way of using muscles exactly as required for each movement. This allows a release of unnecessary muscular tension. More fundamentally, however, tai chi challenges the basis of the stress

response, teaching people to relax the body instead of tensing in stressful situations. This is a major benefit of partnerwork (see pages 148–51). By repeatedly giving and receiving a push, each partner is offered an opportunity to transform the tension it raises into an alert and dynamic relaxation. With training they discover that a more effective way of dealing with a push is to embrace it rather than deny it. The practice strengthens mental and physical confidence, so that body and mind become reprogramed. In time, they react with the fight-or-flight response only in moments of real danger, and the overall level of tension in the body falls significantly.

With so much emphasis on relaxation it is easy to misunderstand the role of tension in the body. Tension in muscles is normal, enabling us to stand and walk, As one group of muscles tenses for action, another relaxes. Normal muscular tension is also beneficial, since in well-exercised legs it will stimulate the upward flow of blood circulating through the veins and lymph flowing along vessels rising from the feet and legs to the heart. The deep veins of the legs send blood flowing upward against the force of gravity to the heart. During exercise, the moving muscles press against the wall of the veins, acting like a pump to speed the blood flow through them. They have the same effect on the lymph vessels, which are not powered by the pumping heart.

Tai chi improves posture and, in time, enhances the benefit to be derived from it. Muscle tone improves because improved alignment increases the energy flow as a direct result of bringing a greater polarity of tension and relaxation.

THE VOLUNTARY MUSCLES

The body has more than 650 muscles, including types of muscle that do not work under voluntary control, such as those of the heart and the digestive system, but tai chi is concerned only with those we use consciously when we move. These are the voluntary muscles, attached by tendons to the skeleton, the most important of which are illustrated here. Tai chi encourages the muscles to work together. This is believed to promote the development of jin (see pages 22–29), also called whole body energy. A posture such as Golden Rooster Stands On One Leg, illustrated below, involves almost all the voluntary muscles.

Sternomastoid: Two neck muscles which independently incline the head toward the shoulder and rotate it left or right, and together help keep the head upright.

Trapezius: This muscles raises and rotates the shoulder blade and draws the head back or to the side.

Deltoid: These cover the shoulder joint and raise and rotate the arm.

Serratus anterior: This muscle below the armpit moves the shoulder blade forward and assists in arm-raising and pushing.

Latissimus dorsi: These large back muscles draw the arms into the chest, extend them and have an important role in deep breathing.

Triceps: These muscles straighten the forearms.

External oblique: The muscles at either side of the abdomen which hold the abdomen firm.

Gluteus maximus: The gluteals are the large muscles of the buttocks. They raise the body from a stoop and they rotate the thighs.

Hamstring muscles: These run from the pelvis to join the tibia just below the knee. They bend the knee and rotate it outward.

Soleus: This powerful muscle plays an important part in bending the ankle and pointing the foot.

Achilles tendon: The body's strongest tendon, connects the calf muscle and the ankle.

Pectorals: The large muscles stretching across the chest. They control the shoulder blade and move the arm forward and down.

Biceps brachi: Descending from the shoulder to the forearm, the biceps bend the arms at the elbows and help turn the palms upward.

Intercostal muscles: These small muscles lie between the ribs and help to expand the rib cage on an in-breath and contract it on an out-breath.

Brachioradialis: This muscles works with other muscles to turn the palm of the hand upward.

Rectus abdominis: Two muscles running down the front of the abdomen which bend the trunk forward or to the side.

Quadriceps: A major group of thigh muscles which helps raise the leg from the hip, and in a standing position straightens the leg and locks it.

Gastrocnemius: The calf muscles have a role in bending the knee and in walking.

Peronius longus: These muscles flex or bend the ankle joints.

Flexor digitorum longus: These muscles are connected to the tibia and extend to the four small toes, which they spread out and straighten. The flexor hallucis longus extends the great toe.

太 37 極

BODY ALIGNMENT

One of the first benefits of tai chi is a rapid and noticeable improvement in basic posture. In a practical and straightforward way, tai chi encourages its students to key into the natural design of the body. It restores an awareness of alignments that enable the frame to function with greater ease and strength. Most children enjoy a natural relationship with the body, but as they grow up, some lose this freedom and unconsciously begin to move awkwardly, or gradually forget how to move in a natural and unrestricted way. Exploring body mechanics helps mind and body to regain some of these lost abilities.

The body needs to have a healthy relationship with gravity. But unlike a building, which is rigid, the body is flexible and mobile. Its frame is designed to enable it to sit, lie, stand, walk, run, jump, lift, and carry, and its postural alignment enables the body to perform its movements in a dynamic relationship with gravity.

A frame is an open structure that gives shape and support. The human frame is the structural system of skeleton, tendons, ligaments, and muscles, which give the body its shape and alignment when moving or still. The frame is not inert like the frame of a building, but kinetic. Each bone has its correct position in the skeleton, a certain range of movement,

and a specific alignment with its neighboring bones, the tendons and ligaments that hold it in place, and the muscles that make its movement possible. The body works as a whole, so the misalignment of bones affects posture and movement.

Stooping and slumping, lifting heavy weights with the body wrongly aligned, aggressive exercise, and tension all affect the body's frame. Years of such misuse can undermine its alignment, and this can result in back pain, headaches, and malfunctioning joints. However, the malfunctions caused by poor posture can be prevented and eased by realignment through tai chi.

Rather than fight against the force of gravity, tai chi works with it, allowing gravity to anchor the body into the earth, working to restore the frame's natural flexibility. It achieves this by relaxing muscles and releasing tension all over the body, allowing bones to resume their intended alignment relative to one another. "I didn't realize I was so strong," is a frequent comment from people experiencing postural corrections in a tai chi class. This strength comes from having restored the body's natural relationship with gravity and from the fact that bones and muscles that are correctly aligned can be exercised more effectively.

Standing Like A Mountain, the exercise illustrated opposite, enables you to feel the difference improved alignment can make.

The spine (left) is an excellent example of the body working as a holistic system. Its 33 bones or vertebrae are aligned in an s-shape and its two flexible curves, combined with the ability of the vertebrae to work separately yet together at the same time, give the back its marvelous mobility.

Incorrect alignment of the frame - the bones, joints and muscles (far left) can lead to structural problems such as slipped discs, back pain, and malfunctions of the joints. Tai chi teaches body awareness, so that good posture when lying, sitting, standing, and moving becomes second nature.

STANDING LIKE A MOUNTAIN BETWEEN HEAVEN AND EARTH

This exercise aims to raise awareness of the body's physical support system, and of the relationship between the parts of the body and their alignment, from the feet on the earth to the head in the sky.

STAND LIKE A MOUNTAIN: THE WHOLENESS OF BEING

The thighs and pelvis meet at the hip joint, the largest in the body. Your hip joints are being asked to "soften" and to open up or gently stretch. Your knees are sensitive to alignment. They act as channels, allowing the force of gravity to pass through. The position of the feet affects the alignment of the frame, which rises from them; and from them descends an imaginary channel that anchors the body to the earth center. Become aware of the relationship between your feet and legs and your upper body.

1 *Stand comfortably with your feet well apart. Notice how and where the weight of your body comes down though your feet. Is it toward the toes or the heels, the instep or the outside of each foot, or somewhere in the middle?*

2 *Rock your weight slowly forward to the front of your feet and bring it back. Repeat two more times. When you stop, allow your feet to meet the earth fully, the weight evenly balanced.*

3 *Bring your weight to the instep. You feel immediately unwanted strain on your knees. They are misaligned and not designed to work properly in this position. Redistribute your weight evenly across your feet.*

4 *Realign your knees so they follow the direction of the feet. This maintains the correct relationship between the feet, the knees, and the hips. Feel it by dropping your spine a few inches. Look down to see that your kneecap follows the direction of the toes.*

5 *Stand upright again. Turn your feet to point slightly outward, and once again drop your spine and bend your knees. Check that your knees are in line with your toes. Notice the effect on your hips when doing this.*

6 *Keeping your legs and upper body still, rock your pelvis backward and forward, then from side to side. Feel your pelvis floating. Circle it a few times in each direction. The pelvic girdle is basin-shaped, a holder and carrier. Feel the link between your lower pelvis and your hip joints, and the relationship between your pelvis and your feet.*

7 *Dropping the spine and bending the knees softens and opens the hips. Repeat this movement a few times, allowing your hips to move and open. Feel the connection between feet, knees, and hips. Your feet are anchored to give you stability; your hips allow mobility. Now return your feet to parallel.*

8 *With your feet planted on the ground, your weight distributed evenly so your knees and toes are aligned, and your pelvis free to move, feel how the spine carries you up through your neck toward the sky. The five bones of the sacrum transfer your weight to the pelvic girdle to the legs and feet and so to the earth. Drop your spine slightly to sit into the earth.*

9 *Lift your arms out a little way away from your body. Imagine your shoulder joints open, letting in space. Feel your arms lift farther out. Explore the movement possibilities of your elbows, then your wrists, then turn your fingertips toward each other. Imagine your arms are growing out from your spine, and make a connection between your fingers.*

10 *Direct your attention to the top of your head. Feel how it links through your spine with your sacrum. Soften the top of your head, imagining that from that spot you are lifted. Feel the polarity between your feet in the earth and your head in the sky. This keeps your spine open or stretched up and down, so that it falls into its natural curved shape.*

STABILITY AND MOBILITY

Here, with the help of three guided exercises, you can develop a practical understanding of the qualities of stability, mobility, and the mechanics of tai chi movement. Let your feet meet the earth. Let your knees follow the direction of your toes. Soften your hips. Let your pelvis float and your spine anchor you in the earth and carry you to the sky. These all-important injunctions are the basis of the stability and the key to understanding the nature of tai chi movement, which flows from it, for the body's relationship to the earth is like that of an underwater plant, which is anchored to a rock yet moves with ease in the current.

Many people are unaware at first that their stability is poor, and realize only when their legs ache after a class. This is because they are not used to maintaining a low center of gravity, or to using their legs so much, but it is a sign that tai chi is gradually strengthening the limbs. The process works two ways, so it is through the movements that a beginner develops stability. Trying to deepen the stance by dropping the spine while moving accustoms the legs to work harder and makes it possible to achieve a still lower center of gravity.

Like all tai chi postures, the exercise in stability illustrated below begins with the principles expressed in the posture Stand Like A Mountain Between

Heaven And Earth, shown on the preceding pages. It ensures that every stance or movement is rooted to the earth center but reaches up to the heavens, with all parts of the body connected in between.

All movements emerge from this position of fundamental strength. The exercise in mobility, opposite, shows how to release the movement potential of the stance illustrated below. People often feel strangely unfamiliar with moving when they begin tai chi. Imagine the movement potential being coiled in the bones, joints, and muscles, ready to be expressed as a surge of energy, and allow yourself to shake and wiggle. Next time it will be easier to move.

STABILITY

This is a two-person exercise, although the role of the second person is to act as an assistant, enabling you to do the exercise. Remember to move slowly throughout the exercise, and ask your partner to build up the pressure very gradually as you learn to deal with it. Before you begin, ask your friend to wait quietly while

you find the position Stand Like A Mountain Between Heaven And Earth, shown on page 39, and take a minute or two to relax into it.

Once you are familiar with this exercise, try a few experiments. You could begin by facing each other, or standing back to back. You might increase the distance between you when you start, so you have to bear more of your partner's weight.

1 *When you are feeling comfortably stable and your body has a sense of wholeness, ask your friend to lean in toward you from the side, gently and slowly.*

2 *Drop your spine slightly and let your arms move a few inches out to the sides, meeting the weight leaning against you and channeling it into the earth. If your partner leans too heavily against you, you may have to hold off the force with your arm. This should not happen, so rest and begin again.*

3 *As you become familiar with the feeling of the weight of another body leaning into you from the side and channeling down through your body, ask your friend to roll around you slowly and lean into you from different angles. Notice how you have to make slight changes to your frame to adjust to pressure from ·different angles.*

4 *Remain solidly stable as your partner turns while orbiting around you.*

MOBILITY

For this exercise you need a safe, comfortable space to move in, and a blindfold. Play some of your favorite, soothing music. While doing this exercise you will be blindfolded, so not able to read these directions at the same time. Rather than try to memorize them, record yourself reading them or ask a friend to read them out to you. Take your time with this exercise. It will probably last 10 to 20 minutes, but there is no time limit. You may find yourself drawn into the meditation for up to as long as an hour.

1 *Stand, blindfolded, imagining you hold a ball of light in your hands. Play with it for a minute. Now imagine the light pouring from the ball into your hands and wrists. Imagine the light soothing and oiling the joints, and massaging your hands and wrists.*

2 *Invite the light to move up through your arm bones into your elbows, bringing them freedom of movement. Feel the folding, unfolding, and turning movements of this complex joint, and its link to wrists and hands.*

3 *Follow the light up your arms and pouring into your shoulder joints. Move your arms forward and back, up and down, and out to the sides, exploring their mobility. Think about how each limb is connected from shoulder to finger joint.*

4 *Feel the light flood from your shoulder joint into your shoulder blades and move to your neck. Relaxing your face and jaw, move your neck in every direction. Then follow the light as it moves up into your jaw and skull. Explore the movement of your jawbone.*

5 *The light slowly descends your spine, filling each vertebra and spreading along each rib. Explore the movement possibilities of your upper body. Follow the light down to the sacrum and coccyx. As it circles the pelvic girdle, your hips join the dance. Let yourself move intuitively and creatively.*

6 *Let the light pour into your hip joints, directing your attention to them and supporting their movement. Listen to your pelvis and follow the knowledge that resides in it.*

7 *Follow the light down each thighbone. Your knees fill with light. It pours down your shin bones to your ankles and feet. Your whole frame is alight and alive, a dancing skeleton.*

8 *Bring your body to rest. You may feel like standing or sitting, crouching, squatting, crawling, or even rolling on the floor. Notice your mobility as you move into these different positions. Finish by resting in any position for at least one minute. Remove your blindfold.*

BODY SHAPE AND POSTURE

The qualities of stability and mobility work with perfect synchronicity in the tai chi postures, which combine correct body shape with freedom of movement. The result is a solid strength and flexibility. Each posture is designed to work in a specific way. Tai chi is a holistic practice, so all parts of the body – hips and heels, pelvis and spine, shoulders and hands – work as one. The movements of the arms, for instance, are part of a movement that began in the feet, and an expression of something that is happening to the entire organism.

THE BASIC STANCE

Although every tai chi posture is carried out while standing, the characteristic stance, shown below, is rather like standing and sitting at the same time. By techniques such as keeping the feet firmly planted on the ground, keeping the knees flexible and never locking them, and dropping the spine, you sit yourself into a stance, and maintain this basic posture while moving. This illustration analyzes the basic tai chi stance, and the guidelines given apply to all the postures. Practice the stance as a static posture often, until you are confident enough to be able to adopt it without practice.

The shape adopted by the body in the tai chi stance encourages the release of stress expressed in the shoulders by relaxing and opening the joints, and the muscles that make them work, restoring the natural flow of energy around the arms and head.

The spine effects the turn, which gives the changing shapes their spirals and circles. Turning massages the internal organs and enlivens the basic posture. The vertebrae work together to turn the body from the sacrum upward.

The sacrum transfers the body's weight from the spine to the pelvis, and via the hip joints to the legs, ankles, and feet. The hip joints need to be soft (relaxed), open, and free to move, so the legs, knees, ankles, and feet are aligned.

The pelvis should be held without tension, as if it were floating, and in its natural position. It should not be pushed right forward nor tilted unnaturally back.

The knees follow the direction of the feet and never lock straight. When the body weight is seated mainly in the back leg, the front knee stays slightly bent. When the weight is mainly forward, the back knee is unlocked, though the back leg is extended.

Always keep the head erect and maintain a link between spine, head, and sky.

Complete freedom of movement is given to the elbow joint to allow the forearm and hand full creative expression, with minimal change occurring in the upper arm and shoulders. The elbow joint therefore needs to be kept relaxed and open to facilitate the flow of energy to the wrist and hand.

A push may appear to be a movement of the hands, but it is part of a movement that begins with the feet and is transmitted via the legs and spine to the arms and hands.

The hands may be held in line with the forearms or pulled up and back, but should not droop from the wrists. In some postures, keeping the wrists in line with the forearms enables the elbows to find their correct place.

While the upper body weaves, spirals, and circles, the legs and feet must remain correctly aligned to maintain stability.

The ankle joints become more flexible with practice. The semi-sitting stance exercises the ankles, stimulating the flow of energy along the legs to the feet.

The feet must be sensitive, alert, and comfortably anchored to the ground when the body weight is forward, when it is back, and while it is moving from back to front or front to back.

ALIGNING THE HANDS

The following exercise demonstrates the difference between aligning the hands with the forearms and letting them hang down from the wrists.

1 Stand with your arms lifted to chest level and the palms of your hands facing you with the fingertips spread about 2 inches apart. Let your elbows hang close to your sides and your wrists go limp so that your hands drop. Imagine your arms and hands are enclosing something large and cylindrical against your chest.

SOFTENING THE WRISTS

The wrists shape the energy flowing into the hand. It is important to know how to "soften" the wrist or relax it to raise the hand so the palm faces forward.

ALIGNING KNEE AND FOOT

In Lifting Hands (top right) the rear knee and foot are in perfect alignment when the weight is back.

When the weight is forward, as in Shoulder

Stroke (see page 97) or Brush Knee and Push (bottom left), the bent knee should be no farther forward than the toes.

2 Now lift your hands until they are in line with your forearms. The cylindrical shape begins to fly off.

3 Lift your elbows up and out to the front to bring the shape back without letting your hands flop forward. This time the shape enclosed by your arms is defined by your elbows, shoulders, and spine and not just your arms and hands, so it is defined more strongly. Letting the hands drop isolates them from the rest of the body.

INSIDE THE BODY

By comparison with the efficient internal organization of the body, the way most people run their external lives seems chaotic. The perfectly regulated systems that keep the body alive give their unceasing best from the moment of conception to the time of death. Tai chi offers its steady, rhythmic movements as a link between the two. It acknowledges the haphazard, human side of the link by recognizing that we are at all times spirit, mind, emotion, and physique. And it reinforces the role of the body's internal systems by supporting the working of all its organs, from outer skin to heart and brain deep in its interior.

If some stressful event, such as commuting, becomes a constant in an individual's daily life, illness may result. Habitual anxiety and feelings of isolation may be accompanied by digestive troubles and skin breakouts. Depression may set in, disturbing appetite and the motivation to exercise. The end result is fatigue, developing into illness.

Although the body's organs function with scarcely an interruption whether the rest of the body is sick or healthy, tense or relaxed, the quality of their functioning fluctuates in ways that often go unnoticed. The health of an organ depends on a network of mental, emotional, and physical conditions. Someone who is feeling good and fulfilled will be likely to have well-functioning organs, and, if that person also exercises and follows a healthy diet, excellent health.

Studies show that the body works best when the mind is content, but we have known this instinctively for centuries. Throughout history and across cultural boundaries the liver has been associated with the emotion of anger. Bile, crucial to the breakdown of fats (see pages 48–49), is abundantly produced by the liver when a person is happy. This sensitive organ reduces its bile production in response to anger.

Through regular daily practice, and especially through partner practice, tai chi can shed light on ways of dealing with emotions. Techniques of self-expression offer other ways of achieving this (see pages 160–171). It is well known that depression can be the result of pent-up anger, and that anger can result from frustration. These emotions must be allowed to flow rather than be blocked. The flow may be generated through speaking, for example, or writing, or painting.

The delicate, intricate kidneys filter about 15 gallons of water and waste products from the blood each day, releasing about 3 pints as urine. They eliminate poisons such as nicotine, and metals, such as mercury and lead (see pages 48–49). According to Traditional Chinese Medicine, the kidneys store life-essence or jing. The adrenal glands, which produce the hormone adrenaline, sit on top of the kidneys, so these organs are associated with fear. This, in turn, is related to willpower. Feelings of timidity can lead to a holding back from life. Tai chi partnerwork is an excellent antidote to timidity.

Tai chi works holistically to improve the functioning of body and mind. It acknowledges emotions as part of the human condition, and as a way of airing them, creating a space in which they can begin to dissolve, opening the way to a happier state. However, in the same way that massage can release nervous tension held in a muscle, tai chi can dislodge emotion, superficial or deep-seated, held in the body. When this happens in practice, it can disrupt a seemingly harmonious state, but having cleared away an emotional block, the body functions better.

Traditional Chinese medicine has always recognized the importance of the kidneys to overall health, as this illustration of the internal organs shows. They are believed to shape reproduction, physical growth, quality of breathing, bone-marrow production, hearing, vision, hair quality, and the functioning of the brain and spinal cord.

SHALLOW BREATHING

Breathing is normally powered by the diaphragm, a large, dome-shaped muscle which separates the chest from the abdomen. Its rhythmic movements enable you to draw in as many as 20,000 breaths and 5,000 gallons of air in a day. If you are in a state of anxiety or depression, however, you do not make use of the diaphragm and other muscles of the lower chest. Breathing takes place mainly in the top part of the chest, and the amount of air you take in is much reduced, so that the body is starved of oxygen and chi or life energy.

Shallow breathing due to anxiety and tension is a growing problem in modern Western countries. As well as exacerbating imbalances of the mind, such as depression, it undermines health. Not enough oxygen dissolves from the lungs into the bloodstream (see page 53), and to remain healthy all body tissues need a regular supply of oxygen from the blood. In stressful situations the speed and depth of breathing change, and the natural, cyclical rhythm of breathing is lost. People hold their breath in fear.

Poor breathing means low energy levels, because along with oxygen, the blood supplies the tissues with nutrients (see pages 46–7). Attempts to raise energy levels by eating more can have the same effect as overloading a choked fire with more wood. What is needed is a reshaping of the fuel, so that more oxygen and nutrients can reach the body's cells. Tai chi works to restore the habit of natural, deep breathing, to enable the body to release energy most efficiently from the available fuel – the circulating blood. The workings of the body are interconnected, and the quality of the blood depends on the well-being of the vital organs, whose health is shaped in turn by the quality of the blood they receive.

BREATHING IN

Air is drawn into the lungs

The intercostal muscles pull the rib cage up and out

The chest cavity expands

The diaphragm contracts and flattens

BREATHING OUT

Air is forced out of the lungs

The intercostal muscles pull the rib cage in and down

The chest cavity decreases in volume

The diaphragm relaxes and rises as it resumes its dome shape

RELEASE THROUGH TAI CHI

Any tai chi exercise can work toward release of tension, anger, or other pent-up emotions. The third preparatory exercise, the Rainbow Circle (see page 77), for example, focuses on healing the liver. The following exercise is helpful for releasing emotion. It also massages the kidneys and loosens tightness and feelings of rigidity in the spine.

Adopt any strong tai chi stance and relax as deeply as you can. Lift your arms as high as you like and turn your body from one side to the other quite vigorously. At the completion of each turn stop suddenly and shout HEY! or SHOO!. Feel the release coming through your arms and out of your fingers.

THE CIRCULATION

Tai chi provides the exercise the body needs to maintain its marvelous circulatory systems. First, it stimulates the pumping action of the heart. It most likely encourages a slight upbeat, depending on the type of practice, so that in a way, to practice tai chi is like taking your heart for a walk. For many people, an over-sedentary lifestyle results in sluggish circulation of the blood and of the lymph fluid, which supplies the tissues with water and nutrients. Tai chi exercise combined with regular massage provide the necessary stimulants to both.

All the cells in the body are bathed in watery tissue fluid in which are dissolved the nutrients they need to live. Tissue fluid circulates in the bloodstream. The pumping action of the heart channels blood along arteries into a network of progressively smaller blood vessels down to the capillaries, the smallest blood vessels which reach from the organs deep inside the body to the skin.

Molecules of tissue fluid containing water, oxygen, and essential nutrients can pass through the capillary walls into the minute spaces between the cells. From there they can be absorbed when needed by the surrounding cells.

All the time, cells excrete excess water and unwanted chemicals such as carbon dioxide through their walls back into the tissue fluid, which drains into the bloodstream through tiny veins called venules. But a proportion of it, along with waste products such as dead cells and bacteria, drains into the channels of the lymphatic system, the body's second circulatory system, where it becomes lymph, a milky fluid mixed with white blood cells, fats from ducts in the intestine, and proteins. Lymph is filtered at certain points in the body through lymph nodes. These are packed with lymphocytes or white blood cells which destroy microorganisms such as bacteria.

The heart's rhythmical pumping circulates blood around the body very efficiently, but the channels that transport lymph from the tissues back to join the bloodstream have no pump. One-way valves in lymph vessels ensure the fluid circulates in the right direction and the pumping action of muscles during exercise keep it circulating.

One reason why tai chi practice maintains a healthy circulation is that it utilizes the body's natural tension. So much emphasis is placed these days on relaxation that it masks the positive role of tension. Tai chi seeks to establish a balance between tension and relaxation. As one group of muscles tenses, another relaxes, and this mechanism enables us to walk, stand, and sit, for example. Heartbeats send the blood cascading rhythmically around the body, The wonderful synchronicity between heartbeats, breaths, and movements, first experienced in the womb, may be rediscovered by relaxing into tai chi practice.

Stress (see pages 38-39) is a nervous stimulus which destroys this synchronicity, and the heart responds by weakening and becoming diseased. The nervous heart is common today, especially among men in some North European cultures, yet there is a simple preventive measure. It is therapeutic to shine a light into the dark corners of the heart, simply by listening to it. Take time to be still and quiet—after tai chi practice is ideal because body and mind are alive, receptive, and responsive.

NOURISHING THE BODY'S CELLS

Tissue fluid containing water, dissolved oxygen, and nutrients such as calcium, sodium, potassium, and glucose, passes through the walls of the blood capillaries to bathe every cell in the body. Some of this fluid is absorbed into the cells through their walls, and the cells also excrete moisture and chemicals such as carbon dioxide. Some of these wastes from the cells pass into venules or tiny veins, to be returned to the main bloodstream. Other wastes drain into nearby lymphatic vessels and are circulated to lymph nodes where they are filtered through armies of disease-fighting lymphocytes. Lymphocytes are white blood cells that help the immune system to fight disease.

Normal muscular tension in well-exercised legs stimulates the return of circulating blood and lymph upward to the heart.

Capillary

Lymphatic vessel

Tissue fluid with dissolved nutrients

BLOOD CIRCULATION

The **carotid arteries** branch from the subclavian arteries to supply the head with blood.

The **subclavian arteries** branch directly from the aorta and supply the arteries of the arm.

The **inferior vena cava** is a major vein. It collects deoxygenated blood from the abdomen and legs and returns it to the right atrium of the heart.

Most **arteries** in the arms have more than one vein running alongside, so that warm blood returns to the heart even when the hands are cold.

The **jugular veins** collect blood returning from the head and channel it into the superior vena cava and the heart.

The **pulmonary artery** takes blood from the right side of the heart to be oxygenated by the lungs.

The two **pulmonary veins** carry oxygenated blood, transporting it from the lungs back to the heart.

The **aorta**, the largest artery, receives oxygenated blood pumped from the left ventricle of the heart and carries it to the arteries serving the head, limbs, and major organs.

The **femoral vein** carries blood from the leg, upward to the trunk.

Small deep **veins** in the legs lie close to arteries, so cold blood from the feet is warmed on its way back to the heart.

The **radial artery** carries blood from the arm to the hand. At the point where it crosses the wrist a pulse can be felt.

The **femoral arteries** distribute blood from the aorta to the thighs and branch to supply the lower legs.

The **great saphenous vein** runs from the foot up the inside of the leg almost to the hip, and is the longest vein.

Tonsils
These are masses of tissue in the throat packed with lymphocytes which attack cancer cells and microorganisms.

The **armpit** is the site of many lymph nodes, which filter harmful cells and organisms from the lymph.

Lymphatic vessels drain the body tissues of excess fluid and waste products, and transport them to the lymph nodes to be filtered.

Thymus gland
Until the teen years this gland is an important producer of lymphocytes.

Thoracic ducts
These vessels carry lymph from the abdomen to the neck, where they return it to the bloodstream by emptying it into a large vein near the heart.

The **spleen** produces lymphocytes and releases them into the lymph vessels.

LYMPHATIC CIRCULATION

The lymphatic system is an essential part of the body's immune system. Lymphocytes, the white blood cells which attack bacteria and viruses, are produced in organs such as the spleen and carried in the lymph fluid through a network of lymph vessels to the lymph ducts, where it is returned to the bloodstream. Lymph nodes filter lymph through a mesh of lymphocytes, Like veins, the lymph vessels have internal valves which channel the fluid along a one-way system, but there is no central pump. The action of the muscles during exercise speeds the lymphatic circulation.

DIGESTION AND ELIMINATION

The energy for body maintenance, growth, and repair comes from the food we ingest and transport to nourish every part of the body down to its smallest component, the cell. An important part of this complex system involves dealing with the waste products secreted by the cells, which the body eliminates in numerous ingenious ways. The delicate organs of the digestive and excretory systems fit into the protective cavities provided by the ribs and the pelvic girdle – all but one, the largest, which covers the body from head to toe and is its first line of defence against disease: the skin.

Soft and extraordinarily flexible, yet a strong supporting structure and an almost impenetrable barrier against invasion by microorganisms, the skin is a key member of the team of major organs which regulate the body's water balance. This it does through sweating. It works with the intestine, the kidneys, the lungs, and the colon to balance the quantity of water taken in with the amount leaving the body, and it succeeds with such efficiency that this critical balance scarcely deviates from an astonishingly narrow margin, whatever sudden changes in temperature or extra intake of food and drink the body may have to deal with. The organs

Needles at Sea Bottom improves digestion by massaging the colon.

of digestion break down the food we eat into their basic molecules, and these are absorbed into the blood (see pages 46–47). The water balance ensures that nutrients needed by the cells reach them.

Digestion is the system that changes the food we eat into usable energy for body maintenance, growth, and repair. Anticipation is the key to the functioning of the digestive system, since digestion begins with the sensation of hunger and the stimulation of the salivary glands in the mouth. The brain sensitizes the stomach to good news about food, encouraging its digestive abilities. Bad news – that the kitchen closed half an hour ago – leads to an immediate fall in the production of digestive juices. The best way to look after the stomach is to eat with enjoyment and dedication.

Exercise is another essential in caring for the digestion. From gullet (esophagus) to colon, the entire digestive system is governed by rhythmic contractions, called peristalsis, of the muscular walls of organs such as the stomach and intestines. Tai chi encourages a harmonizing of all the body's rhythms, including the rhythms of peristalsis. The colon (large intestine) is especially susceptible to disturbances of its natural rhythm which cause complaints such as irritable bowel syndrome (IBS), in which the colon is affected by spasms. In particular, exercises and postures which involve squatting massage the colon directly, encouraging normal peristaltic movements. Similarly, with the repeated turning of the spine in tai chi

postures, first one way, then the other, the kidneys receive a continual massage. The kidneys are accorded great importance in Traditional Chinese Medicine (see page (44)). They hang either side of the spine relatively loosely, so they respond to movements of the body. As the spine turns to the left, the left-hand kidney is slightly compressed while the right kidney is opened. With the returning move the right-hand kidney is slightly compressed, which causes it to release blood while the left kidney opens to pull in fresh blood. In this way, tai chi takes especial care of this delicate organ of fundamental importance to the body's health.

Digestion is a complex process which continues long after we finish eating and while we sleep. It is strongly influenced by emotions. Appetite loss is often an early sign of emotional disturbance. Tai chi relieves the stress which can have a catastrophic effect on the harmonious working of these essential bodily processes. Its generally calming influence on the body as a whole reduces the cause of spasms and dysfunctions, and encourages the organs of digestion and elimination to function normally.

THE SKIN

The skin regulates the body's water balance by sweating. Each day large quantities of water containing traces of salt and other chemicals are excreted through the sweat glands buried deep in the skin. The steady build-up of heat generated through tai chi exercise opens the pores of the skin, assisting this eliminative process. Sweat on the skin surface cools the body when it is too hot.

DIGESTION

Digestion begins as food enters the mouth, where the process of breakdown starts. Digestion is both a physical and a chemical process in that the food is cut up by the teeth and churned by the stomach and the muscular movements of the gut. At the same time, however, it is broken down by chemicals released at different stages in the digestive process.

In addition to the frontline organs of digestion, illustrated here – the stomach, liver, and small intestine – the lungs play an indirect role in digestion. By supplying oxygen, they allow the fire of the digestive system to burn and so release energy. Along with the colon and kidneys, they also have a role in elimination and in maintaining the body's water balance, since water vapor is released with every out-breath.

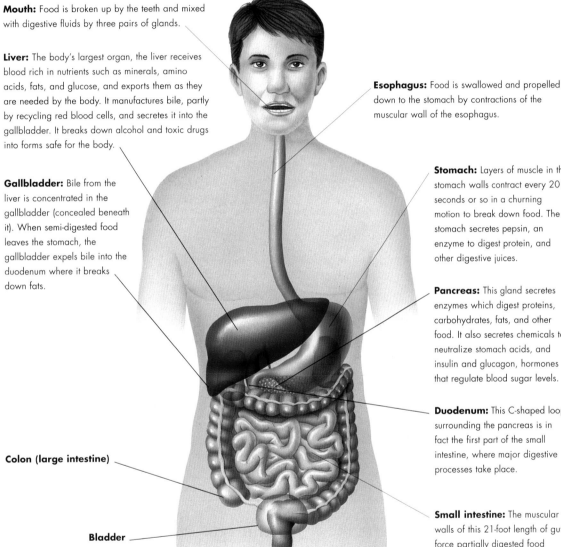

Mouth: Food is broken up by the teeth and mixed with digestive fluids by three pairs of glands.

Liver: The body's largest organ, the liver receives blood rich in nutrients such as minerals, amino acids, fats, and glucose, and exports them as they are needed by the body. It manufactures bile, partly by recycling red blood cells, and secretes it into the gallbladder. It breaks down alcohol and toxic drugs into forms safe for the body.

Gallbladder: Bile from the liver is concentrated in the gallbladder (concealed beneath it). When semi-digested food leaves the stomach, the gallbladder expels bile into the duodenum where it breaks down fats.

Colon (large intestine)

Bladder

Esophagus: Food is swallowed and propelled down to the stomach by contractions of the muscular wall of the esophagus.

Stomach: Layers of muscle in the stomach walls contract every 20 seconds or so in a churning motion to break down food. The stomach secretes pepsin, an enzyme to digest protein, and other digestive juices.

Pancreas: This gland secretes enzymes which digest proteins, carbohydrates, fats, and other food. It also secretes chemicals to neutralize stomach acids, and insulin and glucagon, hormones that regulate blood sugar levels.

Duodenum: This C-shaped loop surrounding the pancreas is in fact the first part of the small intestine, where major digestive processes take place.

Small intestine: The muscular walls of this 21-foot length of gut force partially digested food along to the large intestine. Meanwhile it is absorbed into the blood through fingerlike villi which line it.

ELIMINATION

Liver: Ammonia from the breakdown of proteins is converted in the liver into urea, which is excreted in urine.

Kidneys: Blood is continually filtered by the kidneys, the levels of essential body chemicals kept constant, and wastes and toxic substances removed. These are sent in solution to the bladder as urine. The kidneys play a crucially important role in the body's water balance.

Colon: The main part of the large intestine, about 4 feet long, receives waste products from the small intestine and moves them by contractions of its muscular walls toward the rectum. Water and minerals are absorbed into the blood through its walls.

Rectum: The waste products of digestion pass into the rectum and are excreted as feces.

Bladder: Urea produced by the kidneys, mixed with water, is stored in the bladder and excreted as urine.

SENSORY SYSTEMS

Tai chi practice has the effect of heightening awareness. This process begins with the body, because discovering how and why the body moves raises the consciousness. Developing new ways of responding to other people as a result of learning partner practice expands the awareness. And as tai chi encourages the exploration of the relationship between the self and the cosmos, there is the potential for the awareness to reach new heights.

Tai chi is a sensual practice, and learning it involves expanding sensory awareness, which is rooted in the brain. The cerebellum, an older part of the brain which forms a small sub-brain below the larger and more highly developed cerebrum, coordinates the body's posture, balance, and fine voluntary movements. Studying tai chi stimulates this area of the brain. It also brings increased sensitivity through developing the quality of touch, particularly in the partner exercises. Each person learns to listen, through touch, to the other. The learning process extends naturally to include the thoughts and feelings of the partner. The hands, which have more nerve endings than any other part of the body, gather information. Tai chi encourages each partner to feel more deeply, to extend awareness through touch toward the other person. In time they learn to read the moment when a partner's push is about to begin, or choose the best moment to release a push.

Through partner practice it should become apparent that too much reliance tends to be placed on the sense of sight. In Asia, blind people train as masseurs, their sense of touch being especially keen. Sighted people realize how much they rely on vision when they practice while blindfolded.

Tai chi training works to establish a healthy balance between seeing and feeling. To do this it is essential to dissolve the need for precise, focused vision and allow peripheral vision to come alive. The eye always follows movement, and physiologists speculate that this may be a survival mechanism. Tai chi utilizes this mechanism by encouraging peripheral vision. Looking straight ahead and focusing on a single object transforms the object into a complete experience. Withdrawing the attention from it slightly allows the consciousness to expand, to include a larger dimension so that although the eye continues to look forward, the mind becomes aware of the shape and feeling of the space either side, and any movement in that space becomes evident.

Spatial awareness is more than an interesting visual phenomenon, it is a survival mechanism, an ability that develops from infancy. Tai chi extends and develops it. In time, people become acutely aware of their personal space and develop a sensitivity to the boundaries of other people's space. The heightened awareness of physical space naturally extends into the emotions. People frequently find they can assess the atmosphere of a room, a person, a building, or a landscape more quickly and more completely.

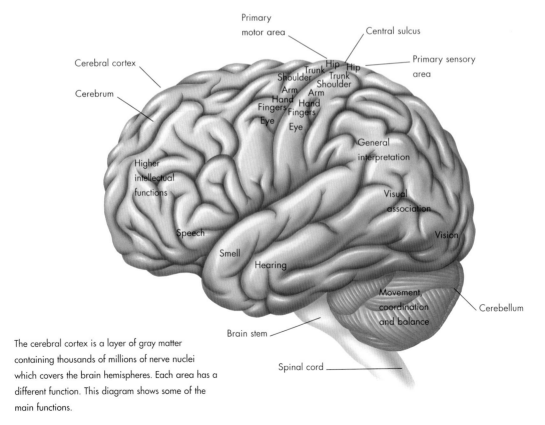

The cerebral cortex is a layer of gray matter containing thousands of millions of nerve nuclei which covers the brain hemispheres. Each area has a different function. This diagram shows some of the main functions.

THE CEREBELLUM

Brain stem

Cerebellum

Spinal cord

The organs of balance in the ear send information about posture to the cerebellum. It is positioned behind the brain stem, the oldest part of the brain, and connected to it by nerve pathways which supply data from structures involved in movement. The tendons, for example, send information about the state of tension or relaxation of the muscles, and the cerebellum controls muscle tone, always keeping one-third of muscle fibers contracted. The cerebellum is called "small brain" because it lies beneath the much larger cerebrum, the most evolved brain area where higher brain functions take place. It communicates with areas in the cerebrum which control movement. The cerebellum coordinates the information it receives and modifies the signals sent to the muscles to ensure movements are smoothly coordinated. It controls balance, working on an automatic level so that we sit, stand, or lean without having to think about how to do it. The cerebellum is capable of learning, so that although tai chi movements may be difficult at first, with practice the cerebellum learns their patterns and incorporates them on a semi-conscious level.

THE SENSE OF SMELL

This sense is a powerful force in human consciousness because it has been essential to our survival. People talk about scenting fear or danger. We have a long memory for smells, and a smell remembered from childhood can evoke deep feelings. Smell directly affects our behavior. To become sensitive to odors, whiffs, and scents is a way of extending the consciousness. Awareness of this sense tends to be masked by the overdominance of sight, hearing, speech, and touch. To bring it to the forefront, the influence of the other senses needs to be reduced. Tai chi practice is one place where an experiment can be carried out safely. In partner practice, for example, you might use your sense of smell as a possible extra source of information. Through exercises like this you raise your general awareness and sensitivity.

Practice identifying smells while wearing a blindfold and ear plugs. Concentrate on sensing and analyzing different odors.

BREATHING

The word "chi" is sometimes translated as "breath" since breathing is so closely associated with the energy of life. It is said that the spirit enters the body of a child the moment it takes its first breath. The physical links between breathing and life are clear – nobody can live without breathing. Tai chi encourages the development of a naturally deep pattern of breathing in which the rhythm of the breath is synchronized with the flow of the movements. This is whole breathing, and its aim is to reap the countless benefits a dynamic metabolism can bring to mind and body.

When moving back in Push posture, some teachers advise breathing out, and breathing in on the forward step, while others say the opposite. The answer is to experiment and adopt the best way for you.

The breath connects the inner life of the body to the outside world through the lungs, which carry on a moment-by-moment dialogue between the body and the space it inhabits. The breath is a messenger, carrying one message into the body and sending a different one to the outside world. This message is carried on the air, which fills the outside world, is drawn temporarily into the body, and expelled from it in an altered form. Air is the element associated with the astrological sign Gemini whose ruling planet is Mercury, the messenger. If the rhythm of the breathing is even, the message carried on the expelled air is one of harmony. Alternatively, sound may surf the

out-breath and travel through the air as messages in speech. Air drawn into the body is needed for its oxygen, the gift of green plants to the global atmosphere, donated over billions of years and now under severe threat from the destructive aspects of modern living.

Breathing is an unconscious process, controlled by the respiration center in the brain. It is impossible to stop yourself breathing long enough to endanger your life. However, some aspects of breathing, such as the speed and depth of the breath, are under voluntary control. Because of the importance of breathing to well-being, many health systems have emerged which seek to develop techniques for improving breathing. Yoga, and the Chinese systems of neigung and qigung (see pages 156–57) are two. Tai chi emphasizes the importance of natural breathing.

Everything in nature, from the tides to the seasons, is cyclical, and breathing is one of life's many cycles with its own natural rhythm. Through harmonious, rhythmic movement tai chi harmonizes the rhythm of the breath with that of the body's movements. It comes through regular practice, but when it happens, a doorway opens and the whole organization of the body changes. It is as if each cell begins to relax and enjoy life, moment by moment, as if body, mind, and soul are able to rest. This resting gives the body a chance to heal, to draw in the vital energy whose circulation through the body we block through repeated episodes of anxiety.

However, there are different theories on how to breathe correctly in tai chi. Some say the postures should end on an out-breath, with the moves between postures being executed on an in-breath. This makes sense in a posture such as Push (see page 93), when the outward movement of the breath complements the outward impetus of the posture. Others argue the opposite, that the in-breath is the energy that fills the posture. The internal expansion in a posture such as Ward Off (see pages 88–90) supports the argument, so this posture, the argument goes, should begin on an out-breath and end on an in-breath.

What is perhaps most important is that the issue should not become a source of anxiety, especially because it produces tension, which inhibits full, healthy breathing. The best advice is to explore and experiment with different ways of breathing in a personal search for what brings about harmony of movement and breathing.

THE LUNGS

Each lung looks like a tree with a cluster of grapes at the end of every branching twig. The grapelike structures, called alveoli, have walls only one cell thick, through which molecules of air and water can pass into tiny blood vessels called capillaries surrounding them. With each breath, oxygen from the air you breathe in passes into the blood, and carbon dioxide and other gases pass into the lung along with water vapor to be breathed out into the air.

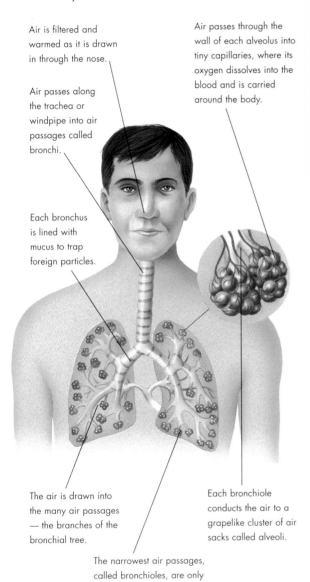

Air is filtered and warmed as it is drawn in through the nose.

Air passes along the trachea or windpipe into air passages called bronchi.

Air passes through the wall of each alveolus into tiny capillaries, where its oxygen dissolves into the blood and is carried around the body.

Each bronchus is lined with mucus to trap foreign particles.

The air is drawn into the many air passages — the branches of the bronchial tree.

Each bronchiole conducts the air to a grapelike cluster of air sacks called alveoli.

The narrowest air passages, called bronchioles, are only one cell thick.

COMMUNE WITH THE SURROUNDING SPACE

You can try this exercise anywhere, at any time, but it can be especially rewarding if you find a place you like, perhaps outdoors in the countryside.

Sit or stand comfortably and direct your attention to your breathing. Watch and listen to your breath entering and leaving your body. Notice how each time you breathe in, the shape of the space around you changes. Notice how each out-breath alters the

From a high vantage point it is easy to imagine the space around you extending to the far horizon.

shape of the space around you in a different way. Explore this feeling. If you are in a room, imagine the shape of the space of the whole room changing as you breathe in and out. If you are outdoors, imagine the air you breathe in has traveled from the horizon. Experience breathing as a communion with the space around you.

TUNE INTO THE PULSE OF THE BREATH

This exercise is aimed at developing sensitivity. It is simple, but you may at first find it hard to focus. Do not be discouraged; with practice you find stronger feeling develops in your hands. Allow five minutes.

Sit or stand comfortably upright. Lift your hands to face each other about 18 inches apart. Think of the space between your hands and imagine you hold a balloon. Squeeze it a little, then again several times. Focus on it until you can feel the pressure. Now direct your awareness to your breathing and notice how the pressure between your hands and the balloon's shape changes in relation to your breathing. Is the pressure greatest on an in-breath, an out-breath, or during the brief pause between in and out and in? Does your body feel different when breathing out from breathing in?

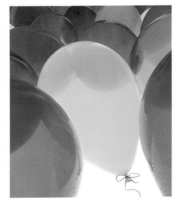

Close your eyes and visualize a bunch of colorful balloons. Choose the brightest, and imagine the touch of the balloon's surface against your skin as your hands squeeze its pliable surface.

THE ENERGY CENTERS

The idea that life energy flows around the body along channels is common to many Eastern medical systems. In Chinese medicine the life force, or chi, flows along channels called meridians; while ancient Hindu medical texts call the energy of life prana, and the channels along which it flows nadis. Spaced along the body's principal nadi, running from the groin along the spine to the top of the head, are seven chakras – vortices or spinning wheels of concentrated energy. Chinese medicine also teaches that the body has seven major energy centers. They may be thought of as points where the chi is more densely concentrated.

The body is immersed in a sea of energy, which surrounds it. Tai chi works to maintain the flow of energy into and out of the body, and its circulation along the meridians.

There is more to the body than its surface physiology. While the many meridians carrying their streams of life energy remain invisible, they can be detected, rather like water holes in the bush, whose location can be detected by a higher level of activity taking place around them than in the surrounding terrain. They have been identified in almost all Eastern medical systems. Acupuncture, for example, identifies 14 meridians, while the traditional Tibetan healing system recognizes many more. And although the existence of the seven energy centers is as yet unproven scientifically, their location is known to correspond with the plexes – concentrated networks of major nerves, such as the solar plexus just below the

diaphragm – and with the positions of the endocrine glands, which secrete hormones. From the energy centers, the life force travels along the meridians to fill every cell. The body senses any changes taking place in the energy surrounding it, and responds to them, so that changes in the body will be transmitted outward and will affect and to some extent shape the surrounding the energy field. Aspects of this energy field, such as the electromagnetic energy generated by all living things, can be measured, but some individuals have the power to see it in its colorful entirety, as an aura emanating from the body and surrounding it.

Tai chi spans the physical, mental, and energetic aspects of life. Like a bridge between matter and consciousness, it shapes and reshapes the body's energy field, keeping its channels clear and energizing them. It opens up exciting possibilities for change to be brought about consciously through working with different aspects of the body. The tai chi postures gather energy and generate it, speed its circulation around the body to make hands and feet glow with warmth, calm its turbulence until the mind rests in tranquility, or send it outward.

It is the potential to regulate the flow of energy that gives tai chi its celebrated healing powers (see pages 24–25). With a rudimentary knowledge of energy pathways and centers, you can harness the power of movement to unblock emotional energy and ease muscular tension, restore feeling, and heighten awareness. This is why it is not essential to know a great deal about the system of the meridians and energy centers in order to practice tai chi, although for anyone interested it could be a valuable study. Instead, feeling the effects of a posture on your body's meridians and energy centers, and witnessing the effects of the changes it brings about in your energy patterns can enrich your practice and enable you to master your life.

The location of the energy centers is known to correspond with the body's main plexes (junctions of major nerves) and the endocrine glands, which secrete hormones.

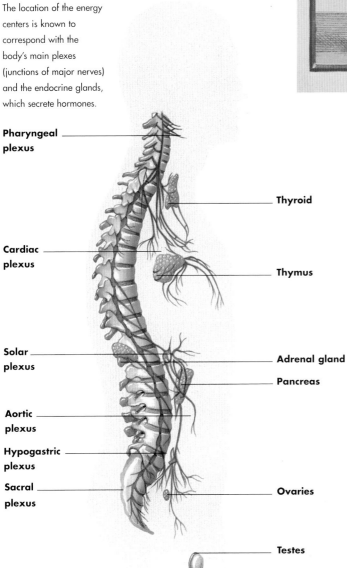

Pharyngeal plexus

Thyroid

Cardiac plexus

Thymus

Solar plexus

Adrenal gland

Pancreas

Aortic plexus

Hypogastric plexus

Sacral plexus

Ovaries

Testes

The ancient Hindu or Vedic healing system distinguishes seven energy centers called *chakras*. Their positions correspond with the major life systems, and with the endocrine glands. The first lies close to the reproductive system and the base of the spine, from where life energy or *prana* rises through each chakra to the seventh, just above the top of the head. Each is intersected by *nadis*, or channels carrying life energy.

Every cell of every type of tissue – bone, cartilage, muscle, nerve, or heart, as in this example – is saturated with chi, life energy, carried along the meridians.

Tai chi acts on the energy centers of the body to stimulate them and to open the mind and body to their influence. There are seven centers, but the higher extension point might be thought of as an eighth. It lies 18 inches above the top of the head, at the top of the aura. Each center corresponds with one of the major nerve junctions and with the glands of the endocrine system, which release directly into the blood hormones that affect the biorhythms, such as the cycle of sleep and wakefulness.

THE SECONDARY CENTERS

The word "hormone" comes from a Greek word meaning "urge on." It is the urging of hormones governing the sexual urges that creates new life, and prompts a mother to begin birthing. Thus, the energy centers form part of an integrated system that includes our sensitivity, awareness, and behavior.

The energy centers are earthed through the root or base chakra in the pelvis and lifted into the dimension of spirit through the crown chakra at the top of the head. In tai chi, earthing is carried out by dropping the pelvis, as if it descended through the legs and feet into the ground; and lifting is effected by raising the top of the head as if it were suspended from above.

Many of the postures in the tai chi form energize one or more of the chakras. The shape made by the body stimulates activity in the energy body. In the posture White Crane Spreads Wings, for instance, one hand is planted down at the level of the pelvic floor and the other is turned up to the heavens and raised above the head, to link the root and crown chakras. The open shape made by the front of the body energizes the solar plexus, focusing it outward.

This interaction with the energy centers gives practice an exciting dimension. The diagram opposite shows how each center is associated with certain qualities - the heart center, for example, with passion and compassion, envy and love. It follows that certain postures might be carried out with the intention of accessing a particular energy center and stimulating the qualities associated with it. If the qualities are in disequilibrium, if, for instance, jealousy is destroying a loving relationship, movements might be carried out to restore a balance. To practice with the awareness of the relationship of tai chi to the body's energy centers provides rich possibilities for self-development.

ACTIVATING THE SECONDARY CENTERS

The Tai Chi postures continually move all the joints of the body and this activates a system of secondary energy centers, shown on the figure on the left. The secondary centers are located on the body's major joints: the shoulders and elbows, the hips and the knees, and there is a center on the palm of each hand and in the center of each foot. It is important to focus the awareness on these points when practicing. Moving with this awareness is like opening a doorway through which energy can pass and is an especially effective method of self-healing.

THE SECONDARY CENTERS

Tai chi, with its emphasis on joints, continually activates the secondary energy centers: center of feet, knees, hips, shoulders, elbows, and palms. Focusing on these points activates them, so it is like opening an energy "doorway". Practicing with this awareness makes it especially good for self-healing.

THE SEVEN MAJOR ENERGY CENTERS

The seven energy centers are aligned along the central pillar of the spine, from its base in the pelvis to the top of the head. The diagram shows the position of each center, and beside it are listed some of the basic qualities often associated with it. Together, the energy centers represent a whole spectrum of possibilities, associations, and attributes. to think in terms of elements.

1 Hui yin, the base or root center

Location: at the coccygeal plexus

Associated gland: the testicles

Associated body parts: sexual organs, colon, legs, feet, bones

Element: earth

The root energy center is located in the sacrum at the base of the spine and fills the lower part of the pelvic basin. It is linked with the need to survive, the sexual urge, reproduction, and material reality.

2 Lower tantien, the sacral or hara center

Location: at the sacral plexus

Associated gland: the ovaries

Associated body parts: kidneys, womb, small intestine, bladder

Element: water

This energy center is located on the lower back (the Ming Men or Gateway to Life), extending toward the front of the body to a point about 2 inches below the navel. "Tantien" means "sea of chi." It is linked with motion, flow, emotion, change, and sexuality. Gut feeling, belly laughter, intuition, and the claiming and establishing of personal power all develop here.

3 Chung Wan or solar plexus center

Location: at the solar plexus

Associated glands: pancreas; the adrenal glands

Associated body parts: liver, stomach, spleen, muscles

Element: fire

This solar-powered energy center is in the middle back and just below the sternum at the front. It allows good energy to pass in and out but prevents unwanted energy from entering the mind/body. It is sensitive to personal power in relation to others, and in imbalance, extremes of the order of ruthless dictatorship and appalling submissiveness are likely. In balance, it is associated with feelings of joyful self-worth.

4 Middle tantien or heart center

Location: pulmonary and cardiac plexi

Associated gland: the thymus

Associated body parts: heart, lungs, arms, hands

Element: air

This center is located between the shoulder blades and the center of the chest. It is a bridge between the physical and non-physical and plays a central, balancing role. It is associated with feeling, honesty, truth, and passion. Every mind is familiar with the heart's uncomfortable, darker aspects—jealousy, envy, and hate—and with its potential, when roused, to pour out compassion and love.

5 Hsuan chi or throat center

Location: at the pharyngeal plexus

Associated glands: the thyroid and parathyroid

Associated body parts: lungs, throat, neck, shoulders, ears, nose

Element: ether is sometimes accredited to the throat energy center

The hsuan chi is the gateway between inside and out, and the messenger that travels between them. It is associated with communication and expression, because feelings and emotions reveal themselves though this gateway. Writing a letter, making a call, speaking, crying, singing, and shouting are all ways of ensuring that this part of you remains open.

6 Upper tantien, the third eye or brow center

Location: at the carotid plexus

Associated gland: the pineal gland

Associated body part: eyes and brain

Projecting from the center of the forehead, this center is linked with visualizing and to some degree with sight. It is associated with imagery, dreaming, and symbolism, with intuition and understanding.

7 Pai hui or crown center

Location: in the cerebral cortex of the brain

Associated gland: the pituitary

Associated body parts: the brain

The aptly named crown energy center fits in and around the head like a halo. It has the finest vibration of all and is your personal link with universal wisdom. Inspirational thoughts, ideas, and profound knowledge are sometimes said to penetrate through to the consciousness at this point.

Each center is associated with one of the seven colours of the spectrum, from red at the root to violet at the crown.

7
6
5
4
3
2
1

3

TAKING STEPS
AND MAKING
MOVES

PREPARING FOR PRACTICE

Before beginning the movements it is useful to have an overview of the nature and purpose of tai chi practice. The guidelines outlined here are an introduction to the practicalities of tai chi and a useful reference to be consulted between practice sessions.

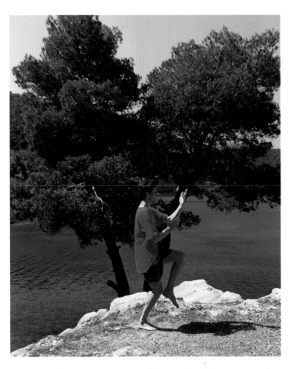

More and more Westerners are following the Chinese custom of practicing outdoors where the air is healthiest.

Practice may take place anywhere, indoors or out. Concentration is important, so some people may prefer to practice alone in a quiet place. Bear in mind, however, that in China, where tai chi originated, it is customary to practice outdoors. In towns or the countryside people seek out places – a rooftop or a hilltop, a park or a garden, beneath trees or beside water – where the air is full of chi or life energy.

Tai chi is energizing rather than tiring, and practicing a form for 10 minutes makes a marvelous start to the day. Alternatively, practice can be relaxing after a frenetic day, making sleep more satisfying. It is wise not to practice for an hour immediately after eating a full meal since digestion uses a great deal of energy. Since tai chi also uses energy, however, it is equally important not to practice on an empty stomach. A light snack half hour or so before beginning is advisable.

To be effective, practice needs to be regular. Although it may be impossible to avoid missing a day now and again, aim to practice for 10 minutes a day at first. Most people find their practice sessions gradually lengthen, some lasting as long as 90 minutes. Three minutes' heartfelt endeavor is always better, however, than one hour's dutiful drudge. If one cannot be involved mentally as well as physically, it is best to cease practicing and resume when inspiration returns. Invite the earth of the body, the light of the

mind, the fire of the passion, and the wisdom of the soul to the feast of each practice.

Try from the beginning to move with focus and intent, not in a heavy, forced manner but with simplicity and the light, innocent, inquisitiveness of a child playing in the sand. This will develop a natural coordination of mind and body and the flexibility to continue learning. It is good always to be uncertain as to what each posture, each movement, will bring.

Books about tai chi can be helpful, especially to beginners, and it is wise to listen to a teacher's advice. But most important of all is *to check out what they say for oneself*. Theoretical knowledge is valuable, but personal knowledge is treasure and students must be careful not to dull the spirit's edge by following theory blindly. It is essential to heed feelings, intuition, and inspiration in search of a personal path. Always ask questions, find out what works and does not work, and why. Never be afraid to improvise around a theme and explore possibilities.

Tai chi practice should be alive. A session may be seen as focused training for living, so qualities that develop there should be taken out into daily life. One might feel like devoting a day to exploring the nature of balance in all aspects of life. Another day it may be listening or spatial awareness. A morning might be spent playing with peripheral vision. At home, at work, or out shopping there is always the potential for letting practice and everyday life become one.

Tai chi is a multidimensional art which can work on all levels of life. Creating time and space for expression after moving as shown on page166–67 is a way of nurturing this.

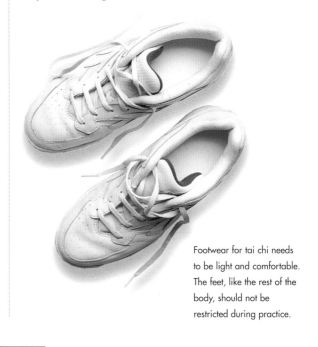

Footwear for tai chi needs to be light and comfortable. The feet, like the rest of the body, should not be restricted during practice.

LEARNING TO RELAX

Before moving, spend some time focusing on each part of your body, so that every part of it is relaxed but alert, ready for movement. Start with the feet, where movement is rooted, to be executed from the legs, controlled by the waist, and materialized in the hands and fingers. Work slowly up to the head.

Your head must be upright. Soften the top by relaxing it physically and mentally. Relax your jawbone and imagine that your skull gives space to your brain.

Relax your face, softening your mouth and the area around your eyes. Imagine your face has an open attitude.

Lift your shoulders and drop them to release tension and unwanted uptightness.

Relax your neck.

Keep your arms relaxed but alert, always ready to stretch. Imagine your arms growing out from your spine, with space developing in your shoulders, elbows and wrists.

The hands need to be comfortable and free to move. Make a fist. Imagine the flesh softening around the bones. Open your hands and spread your fingers.

Soften (depress) the chest to let the chi to sink to the lower tantien.

Relax your elbows so they fall into a natural position.

Drop the base of your spine into the earth while lifting the upper spine through your neck and your head. Imagine space growing between each vertebra. Imagine your spine extending right across your back and the upper part into your arms.

Check that your knees follow the direction of your feet, now and during practice.

Let your hip joints move freely. Feel how they can open and close.

Your feet are the link with the earth on which practice is built. Soften and relax them to allow maximum contact with the ground.

WHAT TO WEAR

It is essential that clothing does not limit your mobility, so choose clothes you feel good in. Natural fibers are most likely to suit your needs for mobility and comfort. You should also experiment with color to find the hues and shades that suit you mentally.

Some people like to practice barefoot, especially outdoors on a welcoming natural surface such as grass, bare earth, or on a sandy beach. Shoes should have flat soles – light sneakers or Chinese-style kung fu slippers are best. Socks can work well on carpet but slide unrestrictedly on a wooden floor.

MOVES AND POSTURES

Although the form is the pillar that supports tai chi, the movements are its foundation. Yang Lu-chan, founder of the classic Yang-style tai chi who lived during the 1700s, did not practice a form as it is known today, but taught a repertoire of moves and postures which he adapted to individual students' needs. The form, though central to modern tai chi, has evolved only during the last 200 to 300 years. Today as in the past, the principles of movement are the heart of tai chi practice.

Maintaining harmony in movement is the basis of the graceful body movements of tai chi.

The form is an unbroken succession of movements in which all parts of the body, from the crown of the head, the face and the eyes, to the fingers and toes move in harmony. Many parts of the body move simultaneously. Just as there is no one definitive form, each tai chi style having its own form and perhaps a number of variations, so do the movements practiced differ from style to style. The various styles include different combinations of movements in their forms, and the way that the movements are executed may change from style to style. In the classic Yang form, for instance, the palms tend to be held open, the hands raised, whereas in the Cheng Man-ch'ing style the hand is aligned with the forearm. The form presented in Part 4 is the Cheng Man-ch'ing Short Form (see pages 84–85) with a short variation.

The form is broken down into what are called postures – although this is a misnomer, since the term "posture" gives the idea of a static pose, and the body is static for a few moments only at the beginning and the end of the form. Postures are short sequences of movements given a descriptive name. Some names have evolved from imitations of the movements of birds or animals – Golden Rooster Stands On One Leg is a good example – while others, such as Push and Punch, describe what happens in the movement.

In tai chi the mind contributes as much as the muscles to every movement. Awareness is the force that directs energy where it is needed and brings to life the spirit of each posture. It is mental awareness, rather than determination, that makes the largest contribution to training the body in balance and correcting the faults in posture that make a true alignment hard to achieve. Movement emerges from stillness, so learning and fully understanding the need for correct alignment and posture when standing still are essential preparations for carrying out the movements of the form.

EARTH CENTER

The Earth holds you to its surface with a loving pull from its center. Through this idea tai chi encourages a healthy relationship with gravity. Cultivate this by imagining a connection from your feet to the center of the earth's core, and by extending feeling downward from your feet. Visualize light beams joining you to the earth center.

REFERENCE POINTS

In the form the attention needs to be in many places simultaneously. Internally, a mental awareness is called upon to make an essential contribution to every movement. You need to feel a connection from your feet down to the center of the earth, and its link to the pelvis, along the spine, and through the top of your head to an imaginary gateway to the cosmos which lies directly above it. Some of the time your focus also needs to be directed outward, for the floor on which you perform tai chi is a compass, providing external references for orientation. These internal and external reference points help you make sense of the movements.

BE AT THE CENTER OF YOUR CIRCLE

Moving or still, you are always connected to your center. Making the connection physical, by aligning your body from the top of your head to your feet on the earth center, gives you a sense of centralized equilibrium. Attune to this alignment mentally and it becomes something that is always with you. Then each step you take, each move you make, each direction you face comes from a sense of balance. Experiencing the world from this position is being at the center of your circle.

The higher extension point lies about 18 inches above the head, bordering the aura that surrounds the body. It links the cosmos to the body and indirectly to the earth through the spine and pelvis. Directing your awareness to this point lifts your spirit through the top of your head.

The top of the head is linked by the spine to the coccyx (tail bone), joining the spirit of the universe to the matter of the earth. Feel it as soft and lifted from above. Directing awareness to it helps maintain a live, dynamic pathway along the spine.

The hands are sensors – they are human antennae. Always be aware of their primary function in tai chi movements, as givers and receivers.

The sacrum is the lower part of the spine that is built into the pelvis. In tai chi it connects the spine to the earth, symbolized by the legs and feet. Directing the awareness to the sacrum makes for effective grounding.

The lower tantien energy center lies halfway between the top of the head and the feet. Also called the "sea of chi," it is the body's battery. Focusing attention here strengthens and balances.

The feet are terminals through which the body becomes a conductor for power from the earth. Imagine a gateway in each foot. All movements in tai chi come from the feet, which keep the body earthed and grounded. Directing the attention to the legs and feet encourages earthing.

The form starts as if the player stands in the center of a circle facing north. The other cardinal directions (south, west, and east), and the non-cardinal directions (northeast, northwest, southeast, and southwest) are incorporated into the choreography of the form. It is traditional to begin facing north. This is said to derive from the idea of aligning with a cosmic center – the Pole Star, which appears as an anchor in the firmament and which navigators in the northern hemisphere use to find the true north. It is not essential when practicing to begin the form facing north, but to follow the directions for the postures and movements on pages 84–143, it is necessary to choose a direction and call it north.

THE LANGUAGE OF TAI CHI MOVEMENTS

There are no unconsidered movements in tai chi. Every circling of an arm, every bending of a knee is the outcome of thought and experiment, and of change brought about over centuries by dedicated teachers and students. Each movement has its meaning, and as the body moves, it forms a succession of different shapes, each of which makes a statement. In this way, tai chi merges body and mind to create a language of body shapes which, performed in set sequences through the form, tell a story.

Every posture involves moving many parts of the body, creating shapes with the arms, hands, legs, and feet, as well as the body as a whole. One way of learning the language of tai chi movements is to distinguish the distinctive feelings produced by the different shapes. Just as sitting in quiet contemplation has a different emotional effect from that produced by waving to someone, so the gathering in of energy during Crossing Hands on page 105 has a distinct feeling from the driving forward of energy in Push on page 93. Tai chi uses body shape to express the mind's intentions, and remarkably small changes in shape can have a major emotional effect.

Tai chi movements carry messages about the position and direction of energy flow and the expression of the spirit. In Single Whip the hands are positioned one facing out and forward, as if sending something, while the other is closed and contained, acting as an anchor. And the punch on pages 102–3 is a gutsy expression of lionhearted spirit.

A STANDING MEDITATION

Every physical and mental movement in this standing meditation is found in the form. As it ends, direct your awareness to the higher extension point at the edge of your aura about 18 inches above your head. You are a unified organism, linked from the center of the earth to the sky.

1 *Stand comfortably with your feet about one shoulder width apart. Slowly rock onto the balls of your feet, then move your weight back to the heels. Repeat several times, finishing with a sense of even weight distribution.*

2 *Bring your awareness to your sacrum (at the base of the spine), perhaps resting a hand there. Feel the triangle made by your right foot, your left foot and your sacrum, and imagine it as your base.*

3 *Imagine gateways into the earth passing through your feet. Through them your consciousness can move into the earth, and the earth into you.*

4 *Take your awareness from your sacrum down through your right leg and foot to the earth center. Then raise it again through your left foot and leg to the sacrum. Repeat four times.*

5 *Soften (focus on relaxing) the top of your head. Feel its link with the sacrum and the connection between sacrum, feet, and earth. Feel a connection from the earth center to the top of your head.*

6 *Imagine your arms are rooted in your spine and that they branch out, opening at the shoulder, elbow, and wrist joints, and into the hands.*

7 *Make a space between each finger and relax the soft flesh around the hard bones of your hands, feeling the contrast.*

8 *Point your hands toward the ground and imagine your fingers having roots that extend into the earth.*

BODY SHAPE – BODY MESSAGE

In the form different expressions are conveyed through palms, fingers, and fists. In White Crane Spreads Wings on page 98, one hand turns up to the sky as a conductor for cosmic energy, and the other faces the earth to conduct earth energy. In Push on page 93 energy travels from the earth through the outward-facing palms. Discover the possibilities of expression through palms, fingers, and fist for yourself by exploring them as shown below; then put them into practice through the three exercises beneath. Familiarize yourself with the way different hand shapes make you feel, exploring your own ideas. Then try different foot positions.

FINGERS

Lift one arm to shoulder height and look along it toward the horizon with your fingers extended. Point each finger in turn at the horizon. Consider how each finger feels. Repeat with the other arm.

FIST

Make a fist with one hand. It should be soft and comfortable, with the thumb tucked outside the knuckles. Play with it, thinking about how it feels to you. Then repeat with the other hand.

PALMS

1 Lift your arms in front of you and turn your palms toward you. Try to sense containment and holding in this position, called "palms facing." Now turn the palms toward the ground and notice the difference in feeling. Repeat the two palm positions.

2 Rotate your palms to face outward. This position carries a sense of energy moving out (try waving to someone with your palm facing).

3 Rest your arms by your sides briefly.

HAND POSITIONS

1 Stand comfortably and think of your internal reference points (see page 63). Turn both palms toward you and try to feel what this shape gives you.

2 Turn one palm up as if in dialogue with the sky, and turn the other to face out – a position called "palm away" – as if communicating with the surrounding space. Feel what this gives you.

3 Drop the hand turned palm away and roll it to face palm down as if in dialogue with the earth. Bring the palm you turned skyward to face your chest. Notice the feelings produced by the new hand shapes.

SOFTENING

"To soften" is a tai chi term meaning to focus on relaxing mentally and physically. Softening the joints leads to an ease of movement and a relaxed condition bringing peace and restfulness.

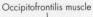

SOFTENING THE TOP OF THE HEAD

A thin sheet of muscle covers the back of the head and most of the forehead. Contracting and relaxing softens the top of the head and stimulates blood flow to the scalp and head. Softening the crown forges the essential link between body and spirit, earth and cosmos.

Occipitofrontilis muscle

SOFTENING THE HIPS

Imagine your hips are as pliable as a child's, with easy, unrestricted movement. To soften them is to relax every muscle, and, mentally, to dissolve internal resistance to opening them, widening their range of movements.

EIGHT BASIC POSTURES

Centuries before modern tai chi forms evolved, the writers of the classic texts spoke of the "Thirteen Patterns" of tai chi. These patterns were sequences of movements making up eight fundamental postures and five basic steps. The Thirteen Patterns are as relevant today as they were when they were first worked out hundreds of years ago, for a sure way to develop confidence and expertise in tai chi is by devoting plenty of time and practice to the basic footwork and hand movements.

8 Elbow (tsou)
Trigram: Tui, lake
Attribute: Joy

Short, sharp, and decisive, Elbow Stroke makes use of the energy generated as the arm folds at the elbow. The elbow is presented forward. As it unfolds, the fist is released to chop up or downward, and its movements can alternate with those of the elbow. Elbow appears in the second part of Turn Body, Chop and Push on page 124.

7 Push (an)
Trigram: Li, fire or vitality
Attribute: Light-giving

Push is a posture that sends energy outward. Always based on listening, it moves out through the hands and like fire, surrounding and consuming the space into which it moves. The fourth primary posture, it appears four times in the form, three times following Ward Off, Rollback, and Press. This ancient pattern of the four primary postures is collectively called Grasp Sparrow's Tail.

6 Split (lieh)
Trigram: Chen, thunder
Attribute: Arousing energy

The secondary posture Split is the explosive force that moves in opposite directions from the same central, spinning source. It appears most spectacularly in the form throughout Diagonal Flying on pages 112–13.

5 Rollback (lu)
Trigram: K'un, receptivity
Attribute: Yielding

Rollback is a protector that delivers a sense of choice. It actively invites incoming energy to the point where it exhausts itself. In neutralizing the incoming energy, Rollback creates a place of choice from where a counter movement or a letting go offer equal possibilities. Rollback, the second primary movement after Ward Off Left, follows Ward Off Right on pages 90–91 and is repeated four more times in the form.

1 Ward off (peng)
Trigram: Ch'ien, heaven or spaciousness
Attribute: Strong

Ward Off energy is sometimes likened to water supporting a boat. It is something that fills the entire body from the inside. It imparts a feeling of a buoyant, natural strength and creates space. Variations on this primary posture, Ward Off Left and Ward Off Right, appear at the beginning of the Short Form (see pages 88–90), where they fill the body with bouncy, springlike energy.

Each of the eight fundamental shapes or postures has its place on the ba gua diagram, and its associated trigram and attribute.

2 Pull (tsai)
Trigram: Sun, wind
Attribute: Sensitivity

Pull tips the balance. Joining with the momentum of something, it adds just enough of its own energy to topple or upset the balance. The first of the secondary postures, it occurs in Single Whip on page 94, when your right hand pulls as it makes a hook shape, a gathering movement; again at the end of the form in the first step of Bend Bow to Shoot Tiger on page 140, when the hands sweep down, pulling something to the earth.

2

Sun

K'an   **3**

Ken

4

3 Press (chi)
Trigram: K'an, water
Attribute: Flowing penetration

Press is like a combination of Ward Off and Push: one arm wards off while the other pushes. It displays a bursting forward of energy up, down, or along, yet it retains a contained shape with which an incoming force may be met and repelled. It follows Rollback on page 92, and is repeated four times in the form. It enhances the bouncy, springlike energy of Ward Off and develops a reactive force.

4 Shoulder (kao)
Trigram: Ken, mountain
Attribute: Stillness and stability

Shoulder stroke is a dynamic expression of solid earth strength, which uses the weight and momentum of the whole body through the shoulder and upper back. The last of the secondary postures, it appears on page 97, where it makes you aware of your own physical strength.

THE STANCES

In tai chi the earth is seen as a living organism having its own life force or chi, so that maintaining a strong connection between the body and the earth is essential to health. An important aim of tai chi practice is to establish channels into the earth through which good nourishment can be obtained from the mother lode of life energy. The legs and feet, therefore, have a fundamental role in tai chi, and to work on their connection to the earth is to shape the fundamental building blocks of the art. Central to this process is the concept of grounding, or earthing.

To be well based is an essential human requirement. Like uprooted plants, people need a source of energy to tap. A tree with roots penetrating deep in the ground can draw moisture and sustenance from the earth, and its stem and leaves can engage in dialogue with light, dark, rain, wind, other plants, and other living creatures. Similarly, rootedness not only gives a person important earth qualities such as balance and stability but it also affects the way in which mind and body connect with the world around.

In tai chi, rooting is a physical process which encourages a condition of grounding. A well-based person gives the impression of having a relaxed solidity, of being in touch with the naturally strong part of the self. Being firmly grounded means that the body becomes the meeting place between the solid spirit of the earth and the cosmic spirit of the heavens. To be well grounded is to be firmly balanced, so

practice begins with techniques aimed at creating central equilibrium (see pages 26 and 70) and establishing a link with the earth center (see page 62). The stances and movements on the following pages are physical expressions of earthing. For example, stepping techniques (see pages 70–71) emphasize keeping the center of gravity low in order to maintain a connection with the earth. Movements involving the pelvis and the lower tantien energy center, the legs and the feet, such as those shown in the box opposite, are exercises in grounding or earthing. And the basic stances, illustrated here, give the body the dynamic stability of a strongly rooted tree.

Tai chi movements can feel awkward at first, but they encourage grounding and beginners soon feel more balanced and earthed. The mind benefits, in that grounding encourages honesty and realism, and the dynamic ability to meet challenges.

THE BASIC STANCES

A movement must be based on the correct stance or foot position. The five basic stances are illustrated below. Practice each of these stances many times, moving the weight from side to side and front to back while keeping the feet still, in order to get used to how the stances feel. When these foot positions occur during the form (see pages 86–143), instructions are given for movements of weight and balance.

1 PARALLEL STANCE

Stand with the feet one shoulder's width apart and parallel (heels and toes aligned). This stance is found in the Beginning posture on pages 86–7, and in Crossing Hands on pages 105 and 142.

REMEMBER

- BLACK: foot is on the ground
- GRAY: lifting off the ground
- OUTLINE: foot is clear of the ground

2 BOW AND ARROW (MOUNTAIN-CLIMBING) STANCE

Stand with your feet one shoulder width apart and parallel (toes and heels aligned), legs slightly bent at the knees. Turn your left foot out to a 45° angle, then lift your right foot and place it two shoulder widths in front of it, Bend your front knee and almost straighten your back (left leg) to give forward momentum like an arrow. Your waist and hips face the direction of your front (right) leg. Repeat the stance, stepping forward with your left leg. This stance occurs often in the form, notably in the four primary postures: Ward Off, Rollback, Press, and Push, which are repeated in the form.

3 THE CAT STANCE

In this stance the feet make an L-shape. Stand, with the feet together, and turn the left foot out at a 90° angle. Move most of your weight onto your left leg. Lift your right foot, take a step forward and lift the heel so that just the ball of the foot touches the ground, and align your hips at a 45° angle to your right foot. Now repeat the posture, moving your weight onto your right leg, lifting your left heel, and aligning your hips at a 45° angle to your left foot. The cat stance appears in step 3 of White Crane Spreads Wings on page 98.

4 THE HEEL STANCE

The feet make an L-shape in this stance, forming a 90° angle to each other, but the toes are lifted. Stand feet together and move most of your weight onto your left leg. Lifting the toes of your right foot, pivot on the heel until your feet form a 90° angle (making an L-shape). Keeping just the heel of your right (front) foot touching the floor, align your hips at an angle of 45° to it. Hold the posture, then repeat it, moving your weight onto your right leg and lifting your left toes. The heel stance appears in step 2 of Lifting Hands on page 96.

BUBBLING WELL

The connection between the body and the earth center, described on pages 62–3, is traditionally held to take place through the point on the foot called the Yongquan, meaning "Bubbling Well." The Yongquan is a gateway in each foot through which you direct your awareness into the earth, and where earth energy can bubble up into your body.

Yongquan or Bubbling Well

5 THE T-STANCE

Despite its name, the feet form an L-shape in this stance. Stand feet together and turn your left foot out at a 90° angle. Step forward with your right foot and place it two shoulder widths in front of your left foot. Move 70% of your weight onto your right leg, then align your pelvis at an angle of 45° to your front foot. The T-stance appears in step 3 of Shoulder Stroke on page 97.

STEPPING

It may seem strange to have to learn to walk again before starting the form, but mastering the principles of stepping is the key to performing the postures successfully. In tai chi the whole person, mind and body, takes part in every step. Here, the complex art of stepping is analyzed, and exercises help newcomers to tai chi to move with poise and grace. Learning to turn a stride or a bouncy step into a slow, steady glide is like practicing scales when learning music. It takes persistent hard work, which is clearly worthwhile when it comes to playing the piece.

The aspects of tai chi covered on the preceding pages, such as posture, central alignment, and stance, all contribute to the ability to step correctly. In tai chi, a step is far from the mechanical lifting and replacing of a foot as most people understand the term, but a steady, rhythmic progression of the weight from front to back and left to right. When performed by a practiced artist the legs may be seen to move, but the whole body from the feet to the crown of the head appears to stay in one plane, in line with the ground, and does not bob up and down. So although stepping backward, forward, and to either side may seem second nature, in tai chi these complex movements need thought and practice.

THE FIVE BASIC STEPS

Central equilibrium (see page 26) is a constant in all stepping, with its presence clearly marked at every moment. Before beginning to move it is important to practice balancing with the feet apart, as shown here, then bringing them close together, before trying out the five basic steps.

move forward (jin)

move back (tui)

The top of the head should feel lifted from above.

The lower tantien or hara energy center is the seat of physical balance.

The sacrum should feel as if something heavy is hanging from it.

Start by placing the feet one shoulder's width apart.

CENTRAL EQUILIBRIUM

move left (ku)

move right (pan)

STEPPING WITH THE BOW AND ARROW STANCE

This stance occurs most often in the form, and involves transferring weight from side to side and front to back while moving the legs. To get a good feel for it, work at gliding the right foot forward while sitting into the left leg, and vice versa. Step 5 is the end of the stance. When you feel confident, go on to step 6, then practice it many times.

3 *Turn your hips in the direction of the right foot, turn the spine, and spiral your weight into that foot. Lift your left heel.*

1 *Stand erect, feet parallel, a shoulder's width apart, the weight evenly distributed, knees slightly bent, following the direction of your feet.*

2 *Sit into your left leg and turn your right foot 90° to the right, pivoting on the heel.*

4 *Balancing on your right leg, turn your spine and hips 45° to the left and place your left foot heel first roughly two shoulder widths forward of its position in step 1.*

5 *Bring about 70% of your weight forward to your left leg, imagining it traveling underground, and push the heel of your right leg down.*

6 *To repeat the stance, bring all your weight forward to the left leg, draw the right foot close to the left and rest it, heel lifted. Step with the right foot 90° to the right.*

TIPS FOR BETTER STEPPING

To achieve smooth, graceful stepping, the contribution made by every part of the body, from upper spine to heels and toes, needs to be analyzed following these rules:

1 Always step from a position of balance and practice central alignment and equilibrium (see page 38) before experimenting with stepping.

2 Never fall into the leg you are stepping into. To be able to step without doing this you need to sit into (or sink deeply into – see page 73) the leg that holds your balance.

3 When moving forward always place the heel of the foot on the ground before the toes.

4 When moving back always place the toes on the ground before the heel.

5 When moving weight from foot to foot imagine your hips are shock absorbers so you do not bob between positions. This places a high demand on your thigh muscles but it makes you feel permanently grounded.

6 When moving weight from foot to foot imagine your weight traveling underground. This helps keep your center of gravity low.

7 Always maintain a good connection with the ground through your feet even when the leg has little weight in it.

BALANCED WALKING

The exercises in balanced walking on these pages put the principles of tai chi stepping into practice. In the form, however, the weight and balance must also be moved while taking steps in all directions. This can be mastered only by learning a number of movements.

When you feel confident about stepping, practice walking in a balanced way forward, then backward; then take several steps to the left and to the right. Take steps of a manageable size, and move slowly and smoothly, making sure of the ground before stepping. When you feel you can perform a balanced walk in each direction, experiment with stepping in any combination you like.

FORWARD

If you resist the impulse to lift your body as you step, you will notice the muscles in your legs working to move your leg forward and you will not bob up between steps. Your feet do not have to be parallel when you step forward or to the side. Take small steps at first.

1 *Stand erect and correctly aligned. Sit into your right leg so you can release the left leg to step.*

2 *Drop your spine and step forward with your left leg. Place the heel first, then the whole foot. Keep your weight on the back leg as you step.*

3 *Check your balance by releasing the front foot, then putting it down, as if testing the ground.*

4 *Keeping both legs still, transfer your weight to your left leg. Imagine it moving underground. Feel the right leg being released, ready to step.*

5 *When the right leg feels released, step forward, keeping your trunk in the same low position.*

6 *Continue to step with balance, never letting your body weight fall on the leading foot. Notice how you drop lower to take longer steps.*

BACKWARD

To walk backward you need your weight and balance planted in one leg and to imagine that you must test the ground before committing weight to it. Stepping backward with the feet parallel helps you move faster and more easily. This technique stretches the Achilles tendon, exercises the ankle joints, and opens the spine.

1 *Sit deeply into your right leg and take a small step backward with the left foot, toes touching the ground first. If you step too far back, you will not be able to rest the foot flat on the ground.*

2 *Check your balance by releasing the back foot, then putting it down as if testing the ground.*

3 *Carefully move your weight from front leg to back, imagining it traveling underground. Step back with the right foot, placing the toes down first.*

4 *Continue to step, keeping your center of gravity low so you do not bob up between steps. Then try stepping backward with your feet parallel.*

THE VOCABULARY OF MOVEMENT

Through tai chi you come to understand and practice a wider range of movements than those you normally use. Over the centuries tai chi has evolved a unique vocabulary, as names have been given to its special movements. "Sitting" the weight into a leg and "folding in" the hips are two earthing movements which may need practice. Developing a connection with the earth is a mental and a physical process. Rather than view the legs as something you balance on, like stilts, you need to feel their dynamic relationship with the earth. The body's weight and the mind's awareness may be visualized as a liquid pouring into the earth; and the legs as channels conducting earth energy up into the body through a gateway in the feet.

SITTING INTO A LEG

Many postures instruct you to "sit into' the left or right leg. With your feet firmly planted, drop your spine earthward while bending the knees. This puts you in a semi-sitting position. Focus on the relationship between the sacrum, the feet, and the earth. They make a strong foundation, like the base of a pyramid through which you feel grounded, yet lifted through the spine and the head. When you feel comfortable sitting into both legs, practice sitting into the left leg, then the right.

FOLDING IN THE HIPS

This movement earths the legs and feet, while granting mobility to the part of the body above the pelvis. Plant your feet firmly on the floor, imagine your hip joints have softened, drop your spine, bend your knees, and begin to squat. Incline your spine slightly forward, until there is just a finger-width of space between your lower pelvis and your upper thigh.

OPENING AND CLOSING

Open and closed are two of the seven basic qualities of tai chi (see pages 26–27), so some part of the body is always opening and closing during tai chi movements.

HIPS

To open a joint is to remind it of its freedom to move. In order to open the hips, stand erect with your feet a shoulder's width apart and your knees slightly bent, and tuck your pelvis inward slightly. Breathe normally, emphasizing the out-breath and focus on relaxing all the muscles in your hips, abdomen, pelvis, and upper thighs. This allows the joints easy, unrestricted movement.

PALMS

This is a fluid movement and it depends on the wrist being softened. To do this, hold your arms out in front of your body and focus your awareness on dispelling tension in muscles, tendons and, bones. Imagine energy flowing into and out of the secondary heart energy center in your palms. When your wrists are fully relaxed, you find your hands move smoothly up and back, opening the palms outward.

1 *Sit into your right leg and take a small step to the left. The inside edge of the foot touches the ground first.*

2 *With all your weight on your front (right) leg, test your balance by releasing the left foot, then putting it down again.*

3 *Move your weight from right leg to left, imagining it traveling underground, then step right. Continue to step slowly, keeping your center of gravity low so you do not bob up between steps.*

KEY MOVES

These two pages present postures in which the legs and feet, once positioned, remain fixed while other parts of the body move. Practiced as solo postures, they offer a fast route to understanding how the tai chi shapes work. Repeating these movements also generates energy, improves circulation, and warms the body. The first three exercises are characterized by repeated turning of the spine, and the different hand shapes show ways of expressing the energy generated by the moving spine. In Push, however, instead of the spine turning, the body remains facing forward while moving forward and back.

Begin each exercise by standing with the feet one shoulder width apart; turn the left foot out to a 45° angle, then move into a bow and arrow stance with the right leg two shoulder widths forward, toes facing ahead, and transfer 70% of your weight to it. (The front foot, pointing in any direction, is the base line, and all other directions are given in relation to it.)

ROLLBACK

1 *Turn your spine from the pelvis as far to the right as you can. The right arm, palm up, extends along the front right diagonal, and the left hand rests palm down opposite the middle of the body and the right elbow.*

2 *Sit into your right leg and transfer 70% of your weight to the back leg, keeping the knee bent. Turn hips and spine to the left, unfold your left forearm from the elbow, rolling it to turn the palm up, and fold the right forearm, turning the palm down.*

3 *Turn your spine right and transfer 70% of your weight to your right leg. Unfold your right elbow, rolling the forearm to turn the palm face up, and folding in your left forearm, turning the palm down. Continue turning to the front right diagonal, finishing in the position at the end of step 1.*

LEFT SIDE

1 *This time, turn your spine left, extend your left arm, palm facing up, along the front left diagonal, and rest the right hand palm down opposite the middle of the body and the right elbow.*

2 *Transfer 70% of your weight back to your right leg while turning to the right and rolling your right forearm to turn the palm face up, and your left forearm to turn the palm down.*

3 *Turn your spine to the left until you face forward while transferring 70% of your weight to your front (left) leg. Unfold your right elbow, rolling the forearm to turn the palm down and your left forearm to turn the palm up. Continue turning to the front left diagonal.*

PRESS AND ROLLBACK

Press first appears on page 92 and occurs four times in the form, always following Rollback. In this exercise the hands join at the palms to press forward, directing energy outward. The movements combine Press and Rollback in one continuous exercise, so that at the end of step 2 you release the press and follow with step 1 of Rollback. Repeat this pattern (rollback, press, rollback, press) continuously on the left and then the right for as long as you like.

RIGHT SIDE

1 *Repeat steps 1 and 2 of Rollback, then bring the left hand to meet the right with the heels of the palms joining as you begin moving your weight forward to your right leg and turn to the right as far as your hips comfortably allow.*

2 *Press well forward during this movement. When all your weight is forward, release your hands from their press position and extend the right arm, palm facing up, along the front right diagonal, and rest the left hand palm down opposite the middle of the body, as in step 1 of Rollback.*

LEFT SIDE

Pause after performing the exercise on one side, rub your legs, then start again with the left foot forward.

1-3 *Repeat steps 1 and 2 of Rollback, then bring your right hand to meet the left, joining the heels of the palms as you begin to move your weight forward to the left leg and turn to the left as far as you can.*

4 *When 70% of your weight is on your front (left) leg, release your hands and extend your left arm, palm up, along the front left diagonal, resting the right hand palm down opposite the middle of the body and the left elbow. From here, follow with step 2 of the Rollback mirror image. Continue repeating steps 1-4 for as long as you wish.*

PUSH

In this exercise the body remains facing forward. The push occurs in step 3 when the back leg pushes the body forward. After step 3, return to step 1 and repeat the movement over and over, generating a flowing, wavelike motion. Push appears four times in the form, first on page 93.

1 *Drop your elbows and lift both arms so that your hands are raised with the palms opposite your shoulders and facing outward.*

2 *Sit 70% of your weight on your back (left) leg and imagine it passing through your left foot into the earth. Keep the front right leg bent at the knee. At the same time, soften (relax) your shoulders, and, elbows leading, bring your hands toward your body in a downward-curving arc.*

3 *Ease your weight forward to your front leg by straightening your back leg, while imagining the weight traveling underground. Lift your hands up to the front and rest them, palms facing outward, opposite your shoulders as in step 1.*

WARM-UP MOVEMENTS

The following six pages illustrate and give step-by-step instructions for 16 sets of movements which make an excellent warm-up sequence before beginning the form. They exercise the body from head to toe, rotating the spine, stretching muscles and joints, and stimulating the nervous system and the circulation of blood, tissue fluid, and life energy. They relax and invigorate. They also make a helpful preparation for the Short Form sequence that follows in Part 4 because they improve balance and coordination.

TURNING

This and the following turn exercise the spine and massage the kidneys, and relax the body as a whole.

Stand comfortably upright with feet parallel and one shoulder's width apart. Rotate the spine, first left and then right. Let the arms swing with the turn and let the weight shift from one leg to the other.

TURNING WITH FEET

While rotating the whole of your spine to the left, bring your weight to the right leg and pivot on the left heel, briefly resting the toes on the floor to face left at a 90° angle to the starting position. Lift the

toes, pivoting the foot to face forward. Transfer your weight to the left leg and repeat the movements turning right. Let your arms swing in coordination with your turning body. Repeat 10–15 times.

THE RAINBOW CIRCLE

This exercise stretches the spine and the legs and massages the liver.

1 *Lift both arms, palms facing forward, and keeping them parallel, paint an imaginary rainbow with them from horizon to horizon. As they fall to the left, bend your spine left and, keeping your legs straight, drop from the hips and continue sweeping your arms as if painting the bottom half of a circular rainbow.*

2 *When you have painted three to five circles from left to right, interrupt the movement on the downward sweep and rest with your body dropped forward and your arms touching the bottom of the arc, to relax your face, neck, and shoulders. Then swing round and up, painting the circle from right to left.*

3 *Finish by resting briefly in the forward bend position, then drop right down into a squat, lifting your hands at the same time as if you are lifting a weight. Finally, raise your legs and stand for a while with your knees slightly bent and your palms facing your abdomen at the level of the lower tantien.*

SAWING WOOD

This exercise encourages grounding and introduces you to the characteristic use of legs, hips, and feet.

Adopt a bow and arrow stance with your right leg forward. Move your weight forward to the right leg and back to the left leg quite swiftly, as if you were cutting across a tree trunk with a large, two-person saw. Let your arms swing in harmony with the rhythm generated by the movement of weight from leg to leg. Keep your hips relaxed and your feet flat, keep both knees slightly bent, and sit your body into the stance so your head and trunk do not bob up and down as your weight moves.

CATHERINE WHEEL

This exercise opens the shoulder joint and stimulates the circulation in the arms.

Adopt a bow and arrow stance with your left leg forward. Rest your left hand on your left hip, make a loose fist with your right hand, and swing your right arm forward, up, back, and down, moving it like a catherine wheel, building momentum to give a lively orbital movement. Continue for as long as you like, then repeat the exercise, swinging the arm back, up, forward, and down. Then step forward with your right leg, rest your right hand on your right hip, and repeat the whole exercise, swinging your left arm.

LEG SWINGS

These swings improve the balance, stretch the legs, develop mobility in the hips, and open the pelvis.

1 *Seat your weight in your left leg, and swing your right leg backward and forward, letting momentum build. As the foot comes forward, point the toes forward, and next time point the heel forward. After several swings, transfer your weight to your right leg and swing your left leg.*

2 *With your feet parallel and your weight seated in your left leg, lift your right leg and swing it out to the right side. Repeat three times. Approach the movement gently, achieving a*

comfortable swing, and you will feel the movement encouraging your hips and pelvis to open. Transfer your weight and balance to your right leg, and repeat the exercise swinging your left leg.

1

2

WILD HORSE

These rotations mobilize the hip joints and develop balance. When practicing, do not be alarmed by the sound of the hip joints moving in their sockets.

1 *Seating your balance in your left leg, rotate your right leg, moving it like a horse pawing the ground, although, while circling, your foot must not touch the ground. Repeat the exercise, circling the leg in the opposite direction.*

2 *Repeat step 1 with your balance in your right leg and rotating your left leg.*

3 *Lift your right leg, bending the knee. Relaxing the lower leg and foot, rotate the hip joint by describing an elliptical shape with the knee, three times clockwise and three times counterclockwise, then rest.*

4 *Transfer your balance to your right leg and repeat step 3 with the left leg.*

CLAPPING

This exercise encourages the chest to open and stale air to be expelled from the lungs. It stimulates the nerve endings and the circulation in the hands.

With the arms relaxed and comfortably extended, clap your hands together in front of your body to give a good slapping sound. Swing your arms back to clap behind the body, letting the breath out of your lungs. Repeat at least five times.

MERIDIAN ARM TWIST

This exercise revitalizes the arms and hands. It opens the meridians (channels of life energy) in the arms, and stretches the muscles, tendons, and ligaments.

1 *Stand upright with your feet parallel and one shoulder's width apart. Drop the spine slightly and lift your arms up and out to shoulder height, palms facing down.*

2 *Turn your left palm up and look along your arm toward it. Relax the arm from the shoulder, imagining your fingers extending from your spine. The more you relax, the more you feel the stretch. At the same time, rotate your right arm along its length, first turning the palm down, then up and back as far as it can go. Hold for at least five seconds, then reverse the twist. Rotate your left palm down, up, and back, while turning to look down your right arm at your right hand which is turned palm up. Look at each finger, feeling your consciousness extend to the tip.*

3 *Repeat step 2 three times finishing palms down as in step 1. Slowly raise your arms with the backs of the hands arcing toward each other until they nearly meet above your head.*

4 *Bring your hands down to touch the top of your head lightly. Keeping your feet flat, drop your spine as far as you can and push up with both hands, turning the palms up.*

5 *Let out a sigh, imagining that you are releasing unwanted, stuck, blocked, or gray life force, while releasing your arms and standing upright.*

SPINE STRETCH PADDLE

This exercise opens and stretches the spine.

1 *Stand comfortably upright, feet a shoulder's width apart. Interlock your fingers, and lift your arms just above your head, turning the joined palms upward. Drop your spine a little.*

2 *Focus your eyes on a point ahead and direct your attention to your neck. Move one elbow forward, down, back, and up, while moving the other back, up, down, and forward. This makes one stroke. Repeat three to five strokes on each side.*

3 *Drop your spine a little more, while raising your hands about 6 inches above your head. Direct your awareness to the middle of your spine, feeling a link between spine and hands. Paddle with your elbows, four strokes each side.*

4 *Drop your spine farther, push your hands to about 15 inches above your head, and keep your hips fixed facing the front. Direct your awareness to the sacrum, feeling a link moving up your spine, through your head to your hands. Paddle with your elbows, perhaps less vigorously.*

5 *Drop your spine as far as you can, push your hands as high as they will go. Feel the link from your coccyx (tail bone) to your hands. With a good sigh release your hands and rest.*

6 *Simply throw both arms up and out to the sides three or four times.*

SPINAL WAVE

1 *Send your chin forward, and on an out-breath drop your head, drop your hips, and move your spine forward.*

This exercise stimulates the thyroid gland, which has a role in the metabolism and digestion of sugars.

2 *Tuck your chin in initially as you draw your breath in and move back to an upright position. This gives a wavelike motion up the spine. Repeat two more times.*

SNAKE SHAKE

This move improves the flexibility of the spine and massages the internal organs, refreshing them by increasing their supply of blood and tissue fluid. It is important to practice gently because the exercise massages the lungs vigorously.

1 *Stand comfortably upright and keep the rest of the body as still as possible while swinging the pelvis from side to side. Settle into this movement for a good minute.*

2 *From the sacrum at its base feel your whole spine begin to come to life in a rising wavelike motion as if a snake that lives in your pelvis winds all the way up to the top of your head.*

3 *The rising energy reaches the top of your head, softening the crown and pouring out like a soothing, cleansing liquid that washes over your body. Shake your body, keeping the feet flat on the ground and making the spine rise and fall energetically. Feel the shake through into your fingertips and keep it going for at least 30 seconds.*

4 *Repeat steps 1–3 two more times, letting the shake continue for as long as you wish. Experiment with slow and quick shaking. Finish standing still, feeling your body working and the contrast between its still exterior and the movements of heart and lungs. Notice the vitality of your cells.*

1

2

3

CLEARANCE

Release and clearance of stale energy is brought about by this vigorous arm movement.

Raise your right arm above your head. Bring it crashing down to stop abruptly opposite the pelvis, and accompany the move with a loud ssshhh as you expel air through your mouth.

Raise your left arm above your head and repeat the movement. Repeat it five to ten times on each side. Imagine releasing any unwanted feelings, clearing your emotions.

DRAWING THREADS

Softly and gently lift your right hand up to the sky as if you were pulling a silken thread from the earth and attaching it to a star. Now lift your left hand, repeating the visualization and letting your right hand drop as it rises. Repeat three, five, or seven times on each side. Finish by bringing both arms well above your head. As you move, imagine you fill the space you clear with creative life energies. Feel how this clears a path from spirit to matter, affirming the links between the part of you in contact with the earth and the part that opens up to the cosmos.

INVOCATION

Raise both arms above your head and feel the space around your hands as part of yourself. Feel the link from the sky through your body to the earth. Invite the powerful, nurturing, inspirational energies of the earth and sky into your body/mind space. Gradually, with your attention fine-tuned, drop your hands through the space around your body as if you were settling the surrounding air. Notice the sensations, feelings, and atmospheres of the space your hands descend through. When your arms are lowered and you can feel the earth through your fingers, conclude by bringing the left hand to rest on the lower tantien energy center just below the navel, and the right hand to rest on the left hand. Rest in this position for at least 30 seconds before finishing.

4

THE COMPLETE
SHORT FORM

INTRODUCING THE FORM

The form – the essence of tai chi – is the subject of this chapter. Each of the following pages illustrates, step by step, the sequence of postures that makes up one form. The approach to the form in this book is unique in that, alongside the analysis of the physical movements that make up each posture, guidelines are given to the mental awareness which, ideally, should accompany them. Tai chi is a holistic practice in which the mental component is as important as the physical, and imagination and visualization make an immense difference to the performance of the postures and their effectiveness in achieving health.

The step-by-step instructions are written for individuals who want to practice alone at home or with friends in small groups. It is scarcely possible to learn tai chi without instruction from a teacher, but this chapter can provide a useful framework for daily practice between sessions, for anyone unable to attend classes regularly and those who have been learning tai chi for some time.

The form presented in this chapter is based on the Cheng Man-ch'ing style. A respected tai chi master who taught for many years in China, Cheng Man-ch'ing transformed the classic Yang tai chi style, shortening it and making it more concise. Anyone familiar with the Cheng Man-ch'ing Short Form will notice, however, that the sequence of movements and the positions of the hands presented in this book differ from the version they first learned.

In the late 1950s a disciple of Cheng Man-ch'ing, Dr. Chi Chiang-tao, introduced a new version of his teacher's form: he took a sequence of movements from the Yang Style Long Form, shown opposite, and added it to Cheng Man-ch'ing's Short Form. Cheng's original sequence is shown opposite, while Dr. Chi Chiang-tao's variation is the part of the form on pages 122–27.

Dr. Chi made this change – as he explained to me, then his student, some years ago – for the benefit of his

Dr. Chi Chiang-tao,
author of the variation on
Cheng Man-Ch'ing's short form
illustrated in this chapter.

students' health. One posture he took from the Yang Style Long Form, called Needles at Sea Bottom, is especially beneficial for the internal organs, and the sequence improves coordination and balance.

There are many ways of interpreting tai chi, and Chi Chiang-tao's variation of the Cheng Man-ch'ing Short Form is presented in a way that is adaptable to individual needs. For instance, the hand positions or "shapes" are true to the original style in the posture called Brush Knee and Push, illustrated on page 99. However, the posture appears again on page 101, this time with variations on the hand shapes.

These variations teach alternative ways of moving, and so broaden experience. A skilful teacher can help students discover the most appropriate way for them. For instance, those needing to relax or "soften" their technique might be encouraged to keep their hands in line with their wrists (in the Cheng Man-ch'ing style) for the first three months of practice; whereas those whose technique is soft but timid might be encouraged to open their palms (in the Yang style) to develop a sense of journeying outward. With regular practice, both groups will learn to feel the different influences of these two hand positions (illustrated on page 93) and discover when and how to use them.

Although you can practice the tai chi form as a succession of purely physical movements, it also offers a spiritual dimension. Before the first posture and after the last one there is a moment of stillness. These pauses provide an opportunity to think about one person's role in the greater web of life and of the importance of the moment as a summation of the story so far in the life of one individual. The movements in the form may then come to have more personal meaning.

Tai chi is not a religion and should not be practiced with the expectation of deep spiritual experiences, but opening oneself to the possibility of spiritual growth may prove to be rewarding. On one level, tai chi may provide a non-religious antidote to the spiritually draining trends in modern living; and on another, it could blossom into a uniquely personal experience.

GUIDE TO THE SHORT FORM:

- With daily practice it takes about 1 year to learn the Short Form.
- The complete Short Form sequence of postures takes 7–10 minutes to perform.
- Ideally, students should aim to practice once a day for perhaps 10 minutes at first, working up to perhaps a half hour a day or longer.
- The following pages give step-by-step guidelines for each movement in the sequence, but it is advisable to attend introductory courses and classes in addition to practicing alone.
- The guidelines given for mental awareness while performing the postures are offered as helpful support rather than as a definitive instruction.
- The Chi Chiang-tao variation begins with the posture Brush Left Knee and Push on page 122 and ends on page 127 with Brush Right Knee and Push.

CHENG MAN-CH'ING'S ORIGINAL SEQUENCE:

Illustrated here is the sequence of postures as found in the original Cheng Man-ch'ing form. Separate Left Foot on page 121 is followed by Turn and Kick With Heel, the first posture illustrated here. The sequence continues with Brush Left Knee and Push followed by Brush Right Knee and Push. The remainder of the form, from Brush Left Knee and Punch Downward on page 128 to Completion on page 143, follows Cheng Man-ch'ing's original sequence.

1 TURN AND KICK WITH HEEL

Still balancing on your right leg, turn on the heel of your right foot so that it faces south, and kick with your heel toward the east.

2 BRUSH LEFT KNEE AND PUSH

Step forward into a bow and arrow stance, leading with your left leg, and push forward with your right hand as illustrated in Brush Knee and Push on pages 99 and 101.

3 BRUSH RIGHT KNEE AND PUSH

Turning your left foot to the left diagonal, facing southwest, bring your weight onto your left leg. Now release your right foot to step into a bow and arrow stance, brushing your right knee and pushing forward with your left hand.

BEGINNING

It is important from the very beginning of the form to work at developing awareness. It is helpful to begin this position by taking in the room, landscape, or cityscape in which one is practicing, noticing the surrounding colors, shapes, and atmosphere, and thinking about the body's place in the space it occupies. Take as long as necessary to focus fully on the present.

The first step connects the body with the earth. It is followed by a sequence of movements describing a cycle which draws up and in, then returns to the earth. There is much to remember at the start, but bear in mind that although the postures appear as steps on the pages, the movements are performed slowly and rhythmically in an unbroken flow.

1 *Stand comfortably upright, facing north, with the arms hanging loosely and the heels together.*

BREATHING

From the beginning, become aware of your breathing. Let your breath to enter your body and leave it comfortably. Notice how your breathing joins you to the space around you. Take three successively deeper, fuller breaths and relax a little further with every out-breath.

2 *Drop your spine, as if seating all your balance in your right leg and sending it into the earth. Release your left foot from the ground and, turning it to face directly north, step to the left, resting it a shoulder's width from your right foot.*

HANDS

During step 3, your hands are comfortably open and relaxed, with a little space between each finger. Your fingers are pointing diagonally earthward, with the little fingers elevated slightly above the other fingers, leading toward the front. This has the effect of opening the back and energizing the arms.

3 *Slowly draw about 60% of your weight onto your left leg, keeping it there through the posture, and lift your arms by drawing your elbows forward. Imagine yourself filling with energy from the earth. Straighten your legs to a more upright stance, moving your right foot parallel to your left foot. Feel connected to the earth through your feet, your hands, and the base of your spine.*

4 Let your arms float upward, relax your wrists, and imagine you are drawing energy from the earth up your spine and up through the space around you. Lift your arms until they are parallel to the ground, letting your hands droop from the wrists.

5 Feel the connection from the earth through the center of your body to the crown of your head. It moves along your arms, and as it reaches your hands and fingers, let them float up until they are in line with your arms and parallel to the ground. Feel the earth energy reach your fingertips.

6 Relax your shoulders and let your elbows drop. This pulls your hands in toward your body. Let your wrists hang naturally. Sink your wrists, allowing your fingers to float and your palms to open, facing forward. Pause to soften (relax) your whole being. Consider the miracle of your life, allowing feelings of joy to fill your body.

7 Let your hands float down, to rest with your arms slightly lifted, your elbows slightly forward, completing the cycle and returning to earth. Let your spine drop as far as you comfortably can, so you finish almost sitting in a standing position. Your stance should be solid and your weight still distributed 60% on the left leg and 40% on the right. You should feel as if you have been earthed.

start position

Start each posture in the position in which you ended the last one.

WARD OFF LEFT

This second posture continues the earthing theme established in the first. Its associated trigram is Ch'ien – heaven or spaciousness – so it links grounding with a sense of spaciousness and displays two contrasting aspects: gathering in and expanding outward. Ward Off Left, together with Ward Off Right, Rollback, Press, and Push (see pages 90–93) are collectively called Grasp Sparrow's Tail. They make up the four primary moves of the eight basic postures (Ward Off Left and Ward Off Right are variations on the primary posture Ward Off, illustrated on page 68). Ward Off Left builds strength in the pelvis, seat of the hui yin and lower tantien energy centers, associated with sexual and creative energies. Sexual energy may be seen as the primal force of creation and the root of creative life energies. Building energy in the pelvis therefore feeds the body's life force and so benefits health.

1 *From the semi-sitting position you held at the end of the first posture, with your weight distributed 60% on your left leg and 40% on your right, your arms lifted, and your elbows slightly forward, make a minor turn to the left.*

VISUALIZATION

It is good to harness the sexual and creative energies during the first step by imagining yourself collecting and gathering between the hands something that feeds and empowers the pelvic area; and during the last steps by remembering the connection between feet, earth, and pelvis. In the final moment, imagine a center of power in the pelvic area spreading through the body.

2 *Slowly move all your weight onto your left leg as you make a large turn 90° to the right, pivoting on your right heel and bringing the foot to rest facing east. Raise your right arm as if you were collecting a large ball beneath it, and support it by bringing your left arm beneath it.*

3 *Following the direction of your right foot, sit all your weight onto your right leg, allowing your left leg to rest behind with the heel lifted.*

4 *Sitting into your right leg, release your left foot to step north into a bow and arrow stance, placing the heel down first. Your weight rests mainly on the back (right) leg. Your feet describe a 90° angle, a shoulder's width apart and twice this distance front to back. Do not lock the front leg at the knee.*

HANDS

During step 3, bring your right hand to rest opposite the middle tantien or heart energy center, and turn the palm down. Your left hand rises no higher than the lower tantien center in the pelvis, and rests palm facing and turned up slightly.

ARMS

From step 3, your arms continue moving slowly, so that by step 5 your left arm is opposite the center of your chest, comfortably curved and with the palm facing, and your right hand is opposite your left thigh with either the fingers or the palm facing earthward. As you complete the movement, note how the posture's final shape feels contained and the right hand acts as an anchor into the earth.

5 *Transfer your weight forward to your front leg, imagining it moving underground, while raising your left arm and lowering your right hand. Push down with your back foot, which straightens your back leg, turns your body to face north, and turns the toes of your back foot 45° to the northeast. Finish with your weight distributed 70% on the back (right) leg and 30% on the front leg.*

TAI CHI TERMS

Palm facing: the palm of the hand is turned to face the body.
Shape: position made with the body or parts of the body.

REFERENCE GUIDE:

- The turns referred to in steps 1 and 2 are illustrated on page 76 (exercises 1 and 2).
- The bow and arrow stance referred to in steps 3 and 4 is illustrated on page 68.
- The action of sitting or seating the weight into or on one of the legs is described on page 73.

start position

WARD OFF RIGHT

Like a wave, these two postures flow on from the end of the last. The way to begin is by imagining oneself gathering the energy generated in Ward Off Left to mobilize it. Ward Off Right is not just a mirror image of its predecessor; it takes the contained energy of Ward Off Left and develops it, giving a more outward expression of Ward Off, one of the primary moves (see page 68). Ward Off Right is the wave racing to the shore, flowing into Rollback – the wave breaking and rolling back into the swell. It energizes the body by drawing up the creative sexual energy of Ward Off and giving it the possibility of expression.

1 *Dropping all your weight onto the front (left) leg, turn your spine a little to the left. Turn the left palm down and the right palm upward, as if collecting a large ball. Your left palm is level with your throat, your right palm with the lower pelvis.*

2 *With your balance on your left leg, step with your right foot into a bow and arrow stance to face east.*

3 *Finish facing east, with 70% of your weight on the front (right) leg and 30% on the back leg. Your right arm leads up and away, your left arm following. This marks the end of the posture, which flows without a break into Rollback.*

HANDS

Your right hand, palm facing, rises up and away in step 3 to finish opposite your throat with the elbow dropped. Your left hand supports it, finishing the movement with the fingers pointing toward the right palm, and about 8 inches away from it. As your leading arm rises, imagine a surge of energy in your body like a wave racing toward the shore. Notice how the movement links the pelvic area with the throat. Feel how the right arm is in the front line with the left hand supporting.

ROLLBACK

This is one of the four primary postures. Its associated trigram is K'un, meaning receptivity and earth. Rollback can receive or absorb a strike or push from an opponent, and offer a simultaneous counter. It teaches how to draw boundaries and hold one's space; and how to earth awkward incoming energy. As you begin, extend your awareness southeast along the diagonal. Become receptive, as if going out to meet something. Be aware of aligning with the diagonal – feel it in front, behind you, and to the left. Let your mind travel with the spiraling, rolling movement, which gathers from the front right (southeast), carries back, and releases.

1 *While visualizing the wave breaking, remain anchored in the front (right) leg, relax, and make a small turn southeast, toward the diagonal running southeast–northwest. Your hands have dropped, the right hand into the position for shaking hands, and the left hand opposite the right elbow.*

2 *Simultaneously move your weight back along the diagonal, rotate your spine to the left, rotate your left forearm until the palm faces upward, and drop your right elbow to let the right hand float up. Finish with 70% of your weight on your back (left) leg, 30% on your front leg, your hips facing the northeast diagonal, the right palm facing north, and the fingers of your left hand near your right elbow.*

3 *Continue to turn as far as your hips will allow. Unfold your left forearm toward the northwest, palm up, and rest your right forearm palm down near your sternum (breastbone). Finish with 90% of your weight resting on your left leg, 10% on your right.*

VISUALIZATION

When you have become familiar with the whole posture, try to enhance its effects by visualizing a wave, which rises with Ward Off Right, breaks on the beach with the first part of Rollback, and washes back down the beach to the sea with the second part.

太 91 極

start position

PRESS

Press is a fabulous bursting forward of energy. Its associated trigram is K'an, water or flowing penetration, and it can be seen as a cleansing posture. Just as water seeps everywhere, so each cell of the body is energized, uniting to give a focused release of energy. Push, which follows Press, uses outgoing energy in a different way, and has a different source. Ward Off Right, Rollback, and Press all come from a pattern of spinal movements involving repeated turns. Push intercepts this pattern to describe a circle from front to back to front.

1 *Push your body forward from the back (left) leg (no stepping happens here).*

VISUALIZATION

Begin this posture by listening behind to the northwest, the left rear diagonal, where Rollback has been released. Do not twist your body to look, but listen carefully, and draw in from this direction. You can imagine that you draw into your body the fluid from a river of gold. Imagine this pouring in through your spine to pile on the momentum of the movement of the push at the beginning of the posture. Feel an involvement in every part of your body.

2 *Anchor in the front leg, and without stepping finish in a bow and arrow stance facing east. Let your vision lay a path for your spirit to ride on, leading directly away to the horizon before you. Your weight finishes 70% on the front (right) leg and 30% on the left leg behind it.*

HANDS

As you push your body forward, your left hand joins the right, with the heels of the palms meeting and the outside of the right hand leading.

PUSH

The trigram for this, the last of the four primary postures, is Li, fire and vitality. The fire of the earth is pulled up through the body by Push, which has a revitalizing effect on energy levels. It can be repeated as a solo exercise time and again, to improve focus and concentration and build life force. Physically, it is especially helpful in developing flexibility in the ankles. Experience moving back at the beginning of this posture as a gathering in. Direct the focus inward and imagine connecting with the hot core of the earth's center. While moving forward, let this image fill the body, and generate a sense of directing the attention outward. The eyes should be used to focus the spirit.

1 *With your weight seated in the front (right) leg, let your hands part as if allowing the focused energy of Press to dissipate. Move your weight to the back leg, keeping the front knee from locking and the front foot firmly connected to the ground.*

2 *Push forward from your back (left) leg to resume the bow and arrow stance and, with shoulders relaxed and elbows dropped, raise your hands slightly, palms toward the front. Your weight finishes 70% on the front (right) leg, 30% on the back leg.*

HANDS

As you transfer your weight from front to back during step 1, your hands are guided back and down by the image of your forearms dropping, with the elbows leading, as if over a wave rolling toward you. This allows your hands to float, and they move toward you when you drop your elbows in mid-posture. Finish step 2 with your elbows only slightly risen from this position, and your hands in line with your forearm, Cheng Man-ch'ing style (top), or with your wrists set back to open the palms in traditional Yang style (bottom).

start position

SINGLE WHIP

This famous posture occurs in all tai chi styles. It can be applied so that it contains each of the four secondary postures of the basic eight – pull, split, elbow, and shoulder – so it could almost be said that knowing the form as far as this seventh posture is all that is necessary, as it embraces all the essential movements of tai chi. Single Whip occurs five times in the Chen Man-ch'ing form, each marking a change in direction and momentum, so that it acts as a marker and a reshuffler. It develops focus, control, and balance. The final shape of the arms encourages an opening and airing of the lungs.

HANDS

Having cast the net during step 1, your hands catch hold of a ball as you turn right in step 3, the right hand on top and the left hand beneath. As you gather the ball in, imagine it to be made of pale gold light. As you finish turning, transform your right hand into a hook (below). As you release the ball of light during the left turn in step 4, consider how one divides into two: the hands move in different directions. Keep some of the released ball's magic in your hook hand. Imagine your left arm dividing an area of light to the right and darkness to the left.

1 *Bring your balance solidly onto your left leg, which has the effect of extending your arms.*

2 *From your hips, turn your spine to the left, arms still reaching out as if throwing something to the northwest corner. Follow with your right foot, turning it through 90°, so it finishes pointing north.*

VISUALIZATION

The first part of this posture is like casting a small fishing net. To do it successfully, you need to focus on anchoring in the back (left) leg, and as you cast your net with your hands in step 1, imagine surrounding yourself with a spray of silver light.

3 *Your feet remain planted as your weight moves from left leg to right, and your spine rotates to the right as far as your hips allow. Fold in your right hip to allow spine and pelvis maximum turn.*

4 *Keeping your balance running from the top of your head through your right leg into the earth, rotate your spine to the left. The momentum extends your right hand toward the northeast. Meanwhile, drop your left elbow while lifting the left hand to face your left shoulder. Your hips face northwest.*

5 *Step west with your left foot into the bow and arrow stance.*

6 *Transfer your weight to your front (left) leg, imagining the weight traveling underground. Straighten your back leg, so your pelvis and torso turn west, the toes of the back (right) foot following around to 45°. Your weight finishes 70% on the front (left) leg and 30% on the back leg.*

TAI CHI TERMS

Palm facing : the palm of the hand faces the body.
Palm away : the palm of the hand is turned to face outward, away from the body.

REFERENCE GUIDE

- The action of folding in the hip, referred to in step 3, is described on page 69.
- The Bow and arrow stance is described on page 68.

HANDS AND ARMS

During step 4 you make a hook (right) with your right hand. Feel how it becomes an anchor and a closed circuit, containing and recirculating energy to the left hand which rises as your body turns, and leads. During step 5 your right arm remains out to the side, where it moved during step 4. Focus on how dark turns to light during this movement. As you straighten your right leg in step 6, your left hand turns from palm facing to palm away, and your awareness moves away as if you were gazing over a landscape. You may end step 6 by setting your wrist back to open the palm further.

start position

LIFTING HANDS

This posture embodies the polarity of opening and closing, developing the ability to open and close physically and mentally. It acts as a breather after the intensity of Single Whip, encouraging deep relaxation and clarity of focus. During step 1, relax completely, allowing yourself to dissolve into the universe. From the vastness of space focus your awareness during step 2 on a point of light like a star about 18 inches from the fingertips of your right hand. This is the place where your fingers would meet if they had extensions. Feel the contrast between this clear focus and the sensation of dispersion at the end of step 1.

2 Draw your arms together while raising your right foot and sweeping it left in coordination with your moving right arm, placing it in the heel stance, facing north. Your feet finish at an angle of 90° to each other. Although your pelvis and torso turn northwest, your head and your attention face north. Your weight is distributed 90% on your left foot and 10% on your right foot.

HANDS

At the end of step 2 your right arm finishes comfortably extended toward the north with the hand at shoulder height. Your left palm faces the right elbow.

1 Relaxing deeply onto your left leg, soften your arms, release your (right) hook hand, and begin turning your palms toward one another. Moving all your weight to your front leg, turn your hips to face northwest while moving your arms into an open gesture. Lift your right heel and pivot the foot.

POINTS TO WATCH

These two postures are very demanding on the left leg. Watch your left knee throughout, making sure your foot stays flat and that your knee always follows your foot. If the knee seems to move to either side, protect it by stopping it from moving. If pivoting your right foot in step 1 of Lifting Hands feels physically demanding, draw your right foot inward after the pivot.

SHOULDER STROKE

This is one of the secondary postures of the basic eight. Its trigram is Ken, mountain or stability, so it expresses solid, mobile power and helps people contact their own physical strength. Like Lifting Hands, it works with polarities – open and close, in and out – journeying from one to the other. As if pulling down from the point of light at the end of Lifting Hands, let your consciousness move through your left foot deep into the earth's center. Focus on this sense of balance, directing your attention inward during step 1. You end step 2 in a new stance – the T-stance (see page 69). In step 3 you journey back from the center of the earth.

1 *At the end of Lifting Hands, pull down. Your body turns to the left. With all your balance on your left leg, draw your right foot in, resting just your toes on the ground next to your left heel. Your head rests quietly on your shoulders, facing west – the same direction as your hips.*

2 *Keeping your balance on your left leg, drop a little and step with your right foot toward the north.*

ARMS AND HANDS

As your body turns left in step 1, your hands drop to face one another level with the lower pelvis (below right). As you push forward in step 3, lift your left hand so the palm faces the inside of your right elbow (as in the figure above right). Imagine pulling fire energy from the earth's center to fill your body until your eyes, ablaze, cast an unwavering gaze forward to the north. Your right arm remains in an arc with the palm facing south.

3 *Keep your feet at an angle of 90° to one another and your vision focused to the north as you push forward from the left rear leg to the front right; your hips turn slightly to face northwest. Your weight finishes 70% on the front (right) leg and 30% on the back leg.*

REFERENCE GUIDE

- The techniques of opening and closing are described on page 73.
- The heel stance, referred to in step 2 of Lifting Hands, is described and illustrated on page 69.
- The T-stance, referred to in step 1 of Shoulder Stroke, is described and illustrated on page 69.

start position

WHITE CRANE SPREADS WINGS

This is the third posture in succession to introduce a new stance – the cat stance (see page 69). With it, the repertoire of foot positions is complete. It also introduces a change in direction from north to west, and it is the first posture to actively open up the dimension of the sky, spreading the body between the earth and the heavens. This opens the front of the body, inviting the energy center at the solar plexus to shine. White Crane Spreads Wings encourages movement out into the world from a relaxed center.

1 *Sink all your weight onto your front (right) leg while your right arm begins to float. Meanwhile, your left hand arcs to the left in a spreading motion. Lift your left heel slightly, then draw your left foot toward your body.*

2 *Step forward with the left foot into the cat stance, facing west, with the ball of your left foot and your whole right foot on the ground.*

VISUALIZATION

Imagine you are opening a space, as if drawing curtains apart, into which you carefully step and look. There is an atmosphere of readiness to act or pounce. Feel the connection from your right hand in the sky to your left hand in the earth, and the connection across your spine from the fingertips of your left hand to those of the right. You might visualize a spiral of golden light running from your right hand, down your right arm, across your back, over your solar plexus at the front and around your body, to finish by connecting into the lower left arm and hand. Imagine your solar plexus pouring out sunshine while restoring healthy functioning.

3 *Your weight and balance stay on your back (right) leg. Your left foot is active, pushing to straighten the legs a little. As this is happening your left hand drops to the left, facing down and away from your body, while your right hand rotates upward, facing the sky. Your weight is distributed 90% on your right leg and 10% on your left.*

BRUSH LEFT KNEE AND PUSH (1)

The ready-for-action energy of White Crane Spreads Wings has a chance for expression in Brush Left Knee and Push, when something is caught and then sent. This posture develops coordination between left and right and encourages the qualities of receiving and giving.

1 Drop all your weight onto your right leg, releasing your left leg ready to step. At the same time, turn your spine to the right as far as your hips allow. Your left hand simultaneously rises in front of your body and your right arm opens fully out to the side.

2 Step west with your left foot into a bow and arrow stance, drop your left hand to the inside of your left thigh, and fold your right arm at the elbow with the hand pointing forward to the west, near your right ear. Your weight is still on your back leg, the right foot is at a 90° angle, and your hips face northwest.

3 Relax your right elbow as you bring your weight forward and straighten your back leg to give a sending movement through the fingers of your right hand. Both hands are in line with your forearms. Your spine turns so you face directly west. Your left arm moves across your left thigh.

VISUALIZATION

During step 1 imagine something flying out toward you from the place you were looking into during the last posture. Meet it with your left forearm, guiding it to the side as you turn. In step 2 it is as if your left hand has served up something for your right hand to aim at, like a tennis player throwing up the ball for the racket. Feel the way your right hand begins to take over from your left. Looking directly forward, to the west, feel how the pointing fingers of your right hand and your vision join in forward momentum. You are now ready to send outward.

Focus your attention clearly forward during step 3, as if sending something with your right hand, especially through the fingers. Feel how your left hand acts as an anchor into the earth.

start position

PLAY GUITAR

The final position for Play Guitar is like a mirror image of Lifting Hands on page 96, but where Lifting Hands gathers inward from the side, Play Guitar moves in the vertical plane. The posture is about stepping forward (and potentially backward) to catch something, so when making the first step, imagine reaching to touch something with the right hand. It trains coordination between stepping, momentum, and arm movement, so the weight moving back in step 2 coordinates with the rising left arm. Focus on timing, so that hands and heel all arrive in their final position together, like something clicking into place. Play Guitar encourages a light, open, balanced perspective, typical of the heart energy center.

1 *Sit into your front (left) leg and step up with your back (right) foot to rest it close to and slightly behind your left foot, at an angle of 45°.*

VISUALIZATION

Play Guitar can be used to develop the energy of the heart center (see page 57). Feel the contained space between your arms, and affirm your connection to the earth through your body. Imagine light pouring from your heart to fill the space created by your arms and hands. Let the light permeate your bones, blood, cells, and whole body, and feel it extend into the surrounding space.

2 *Transfer all your weight to your back (right) leg while extending your left arm so that the hand is at shoulder height and the elbow relaxed downward. Meanwhile, release your left foot to rest the heel a little forward and left of your right foot. Your right hand moves in and downward, resting opposite your left elbow. Finish with your hips facing northwest and 90% of your weight on your back (right) foot and 10% on your front foot.*

BRUSH LEFT KNEE AND PUSH (2)

The version of Brush Knee and Push on this page is similar to that on page 99, but it starts from a quieter place and makes use of the palms of the hands. Instead of catching something flying, as after White Crane Spreads Wings, imagine carrying back the light, open attitude of the last posture – the energy built up during Play Guitar is guided back by the left hand at the beginning of Brush Left Knee and sent out and forward by the right hand.

2 *Step to the west with your left foot in preparation for a bow and arrow stance, drop your left hand to the inside of your left thigh, and fold your right arm at the elbow with the hand pointing forward, to the west, near your right ear. Your weight is still on your back (right) leg and your hips face northwest.*

1 *Keeping your weight on your back (right) leg, with your left hand at chest height, drop your left elbow, folding in your arm a little. Keep your shoulder relaxed while sitting back and turning to the right as far as your hips allow.*

3 *Relax your right elbow as you bring your weight forward and straighten your back leg to give a sending movement through the palm of your right hand, which faces forward, while the left palm faces the earth. Both palms are now open, the right palm facing forward and the left facing the earth.*

太 101 極

start position

PUNCH (1)

The full name for this posture is Step Forward, Deflect Downward, Intercept, and Punch. Gathering root power, it moves into an earthy, heartfelt crescendo with the punch at the end. The use of the fist and the atmosphere of the final posture make a statement in the form. Punch is a gutsy posture, wonderful for coordination and balance, and it is a fine remedy for faintheartedness and a tentative approach to life.

Punch is a coordinated movement that begins in the feet and involves the whole body. The energy is not discharged, but held.

1 *Bring most of your weight onto your back (right) leg, soften (relax) your left hand, and, making a fist of your right hand, move your right arm down to mirror the left. Pivoting on your left heel, turn your left foot to face the front left (southwest) diagonal, and rest it flat.*

POINTS TO WATCH

You make a fist at the end of step 1, and you begin step 3 by making a big turn of almost 180° from south to northwest, which is expressed as a sweeping movement with the right, fist arm. The punch, in step 6, is expressed in the arm, which must be relaxed so that the form of the posture is fluid and fluent. Put your body, feeling, heart, and soul into the punch.

2 *Follow the direction of your left foot with your pelvis and bring all your weight to sit into your left leg. Lift your right heel as your right leg rests behind.*

3 *Relax your spine to the left to give momentum, lift your right foot, and rotate your spine to the right. Halfway through the turn, place your right foot on the ground, heel to the front of the left instep, about 12 inches in front of the toes of your left foot. Your right toes point right (northwest).*

LIGHT SPIRIT

As you make the turn in step 3, the weight of your body spirals down through your right foot into the earth. You seat your balance in your right leg, but this downward force is countered by an upward movement, as if you were suspended from above. The Chinese call this tension between opposite poles "light spirit."

THE FIST IN TAI CHI

It is important to form the fist correctly for tai chi practice. It should not be tense or tight, but soft, yet firm. The thumb bends at the joints, running across the outside of the last set of finger knuckles. The fingers must never curl around the thumb, since in a strike the thumb in this position could break.

The correct mental attitude to the fist is important. When you form a fist during step 1, feel yourself connecting with the physically strong, earthy part of yourself and the hui yin energy center in the pelvis, and gather this feeling in.

4 *Turn your hips in the direction of your right foot, so your trunk faces northwest. Continue turning right and bring all your weight to your right foot, imagining it spiraling through your foot into the earth. Your left foot, heel raised, rests behind.*

5 *Release your left foot to step forward and change your focus to the front (west), looking past your left hand.*

6 *Pushing from your back leg into the bow and arrow stance, release your fist to spiral up and forward, finishing opposite your right shoulder. Finish with your weight distributed 70% on your front (left) leg and 30% on the back (right) leg.*

HANDS

From the beginning of the turn in step 3, sweep your right fist, hand upward, in an arc to drop down by your hip (as photograph right).

Raise your left hand to coordinate with it, so that as your hip drops, your left palm faces the right front (northwest) diagonal. Your right hand, if you opened your fist, would face palm up. Follow this direction with your face and your eyes.

The root energy you gathered as you made a fist during step 1 is employed in step 3 in painting the arc with your fist to link root (lower pelvis) to heart and back to root. Feel the stored power in your fist, and notice how your left hand emerges forward from the tail of this arc of power. Finish step 3 focusing toward the diagonal, eyes and left palm working together, and a clear alignment through your right side.

Moving forward in step 5 brings the left hand closer to the body. It finishes opposite your right elbow, palm facing, and forward from the center of the chest (right).

start position

WITHDRAW AND PUSH

Withdraw and Push releases the energy of the punch at the end of the last posture in a beautiful gesture, then clears the space and fills it again, to give a new start. The posture is sometimes called Apparent Close Up because the body forms a closed-up shape. It teaches the mental and physical aspects of the qualities of full and empty. Feel the contrast between the fullness of the punch at the end of the last posture and the sense of release as you relax your fist hand in step 1. Release your fist gently, as if sending dandelion seeds into the wind.

1 *Sitting into your left hip, turn a little to the left. Simultaneously release your fist, turning the palm of your right hand up slightly. Bring the left hand down, rotating the palm up, until the fingers lie just under your right elbow.*

2 *Bring the weight back onto your right leg and turning to the right, draw your right arm over your left hand as if clearing something from the forearm. Your hips now face northwest. Turn to the west and drop your left elbow so both arms are relaxed, with the palms at stomach height, turned up toward your face.*

3 *Relax your elbows, turn your palms comfortably forward, and imagine you fill the empty space created as you push forward (keeping your feet still) with renewed energy and a sense of a fresh start. Finish with your palms opposite your shoulders.*

VISUALIZATION

In step 2 the sensation of release generated in step 1 turns into a feeling of emptiness. Try to enhance this as if you are the living embodiment of emptiness. Before you push during step 3, imagine you have cleared the space in front of you, then fill that space with the push.

CROSSING HANDS

These movements express a gathering in. Enjoy the openness of the large arm movement in step 2, and be aware of the strong, contained shape you make. Standing in this position for a few minutes as a static posture improves circulation, especially to the arms and hands, and strengthens the back. In a martial sense this is a defensive posture – the crossed hands protect the throat and the front of the body. It reaffirms a condition of central equilibrium, balance, and alignment – the body is anchored in the earth and lifted to the sky.

1 *Leave the fingertips of both hands in their position at the end of Withdraw and Push. Draw your weight onto your right leg. This has the effect of extending the arms forward.*

2 *Fold in your hip and make a 90° turn to the right (north). Bring the toes of your left foot round to face north. Open your arms in a broad arc, palms facing north.*

3 *Coordinate the weight returning to the left leg with a gathering of the arms, which rotate from the elbows to finish palms facing. Step back with your right foot to bring it a shoulder's width from and parallel to the left, as the right palm crosses outside the left and the wrists meet. The palms finish opposite the throat, and the arms create a round space in which energy circulates. Your weight finishes 60% on the left leg and 40% on the right.*

start position

EMBRACE TIGER, RETURN TO MOUNTAIN

Justifying its poetic name and powerful image, Embrace Tiger, Return to Mountain is a dynamic posture. As if responding to an imaginary attack from behind and to the right, the player is called upon to move fearlessly into the path of danger to deal with it. Considering the martial application can be helpful to the performance of this posture, as it gives meaning to the turn, parry, and strike. Its physical benefits are that it develops balance and mobility and opens the hips and groin.

1 *Sit into your left leg, dropping your right hand and turning it palm down and out. Simultaneously lift your right heel and turn right toward the northeast diagonal. Your left arm remains palm facing. Direct your attention behind you to the right.*

VISUALIZATION

During step 1, imagine you contact something with your right palm and the underside of your right forearm. As step 2 begins you take a large step into the path of danger, and in step 3 your right arm averts it, circles, and with the left palm squeezes and pushes the threat away. Feel the link between your palms and between your body, the energy surrounding it, the lower pelvis and the throat. Allow your mind and energy to move outward.

3 *Bring your weight forward while drawing a generous cup shape in the air with your right hand, turning it palm up near your right thigh. Drop your left elbow, turning the hand palm forward, but keeping it level with your throat.*

2 *Take a big step with your right foot, swinging it round to place it heel first in a bow and arrow stance on the southeast diagonal. Your right arm moves with your right leg as if attached to it. Almost all your weight remains on the back (left) leg.*

POINTS TO WATCH

This is the first posture to align along a diagonal, so from the beginning keep your attention on your orientation along the northwest–southeast diagonal. If it is hard to take a big step in step 2, rest your right foot briefly on the ground and use it to balance as you turn your left heel inward at a 45° angle. Bring all your weight to your left leg.

ROLLBACK, PRESS, PUSH, AND SINGLE WHIP

This sequence marks a changeover from one section of the form to another. The same movements are followed as shown on pages 91–5, but the external reference points have changed from the east–west axis to the northwest–southeast diagonal.

ROLLBACK

Here the move into Rollback differs from the version on page 91. Following step 3 of Embrace Tiger, Return to Mountain you make a small adjustment movement before progressing smoothly into step 2 and then step 3 of Rollback on page 91, aligned on the northwest–southeast diagonal.

ADJUSTMENT MOVEMENT

1 *With your weight on your front (right) leg, turn to the right (south), lifting your right palm in an arc and bringing your left palm down opposite your right elbow. Focus southward, in following your arms.*

2 *Simultaneously move your weight back along the diagonal, turn your spine left, rotate your left forearm to turn the palms up, and drop your right elbow to lift the hand. Finish with 70% of your weight on your back (left) leg, hips and right palm facing east, and your left fingers near your right elbow.*

3 *Continue to turn left as far as your hips will allow. Unfold your left forearm toward the north, palm up, and rest your right forearm palm down near your breastbone. Finish with 90% of your weight resting on your left leg, 10% on your right.*

PRESS

Now move smoothly into Press, following the same sequence of movements as shown on page 92, but along the diagonal.

PUSH

Progress without a break into Push, as shown on page 93, but aligning along the diagonal.

SINGLE WHIP

Glide into Single Whip as shown on pages 94–5. Finish on the diagonal, facing northwest. Pay particular attention to the final step, making sure you face the northwest diagonal and do not step all the way round to the west.

start position

PUNCH UNDER ELBOW

Through deft footwork this posture teaches poise, clarity, mobility, and balance in stepping. It develops warrior energy by bridging inner-centeredness with outward focus. After it you feel you can meet anything that comes your way. Through the posture, but especially in step 4, too many movements seem to be taking place at once. Focus on coordinating the movements and all quickly become part of a delightful whirl. At the end, focus awareness on central balance and enjoy feeling poised and focused. Allow awareness to shine out through the eyes.

1 *Sit your weight into your back (right) leg, and step across with your left foot, your left arm traveling with it, as if attached by a thread. Finish with the left foot and left palm facing west.*

POINTS TO WATCH

As you move into step 1, transfer your attention from the diagonal to the front, now west. Your right hand still forms a hook shape. In step 2, focus on your weight pouring into the earth through your left leg – your anchor – while enjoying the turn to the left. Managing the coordination between stepping, weight transfer, and the complex movements of arms, hands, and fingers is the central task in steps 3 and 4. The posture finishes as your left heel meets the earth.

2 *Release your hook hand while moving your weight to your left leg. Keeping your left foot on the ground, turn your spine to the left. Imagine the weight spiraling into the earth through this anchored foot. Step up (west) with your right foot, placing your toes in line with and about 12 inches to the right of the left instep. Your right arm extends west, palm facing south. Drop your left elbow, turning your left palm to face southeast.*

3 *Step back (toward the east) with your right foot, turning your toes northwest and keeping most of your weight on your left (front) foot.*

ARMS AND HANDS

Lift your left elbow in step 3, point the hand downward, and scoop it palm up next to your left hip. Your right hand moves nearer your body to lie palm down opposite the center of your chest. As your weight moves back during step 4, coordinate it with the movement of your left arm, dropping the elbow to raise the arm so that your forearm finishes almost vertical, your fingers pointing to the sky. At the same time, make a fist of your right hand, resting it, as the illustration shows, opposite the solar plexus. As the posture ends, your right forearm is parallel to the ground and if you open your fist, the palm faces the earth.

4 *Transferring all your weight to your back (right) leg, step into a heel stance, placing your left heel forward of the right foot. Your weight finishes 90% on your back (right) leg and 10% on your left leg.*

REFERENCE GUIDE

- The heel stance is illustrated on page 69.

start position

STEP BACK TO REPULSE MONKEY

This spirited move teaches the skill needed to keep one's presence forward while moving physically backward. It involves testing the ground before moving the weight, and keeping a forward eye on the advancing and unpredictable imaginary monkey. It draws on the focused warrior energy of Punch Under Elbow. This posture opens the ankle joints and exercises the Achilles tendons, which helps develop the balance and coordination needed to move backward. It reaffirms the spine's natural alignment and so lifts and sharpens the spirit and heightens awareness. This posture is performed three times, first turning to the right, then to the left, then right.

RIGHT SIDE

Expect to struggle with the difficult coordination in this posture, particularly in step 2 where several movements happen at once. Allow your body to find its own coordination. By contrast with the open shape of step 1, the body is more gathered or closed in step 2.

1 *Keeping your weight mainly on your right (back) leg and your feet still, turn your spine to the right as far as your hips allow. Extend your left arm forward (west), palm down. Release the fist as you drop your right arm, then arc it up and out to the side with the palm facing forward.*

HEAD AND EYES

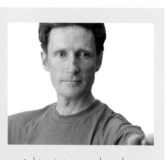

In step 1 there are two possible positions for the head and neck, and three for the eyes. As you turn, you might rotate your head to face west (above) and focus your eyes sharply forward. Since your hips are turned to the north, this exercises your spine and neck. Alternatively, align your head with your body, extending your feeling strongly along the forward arm – the left one in the right-orientated version of the posture and vice versa – and use peripheral vision. You might also keep your head in line with your body and direct your eyes toward the front (west).

VISUALIZATION

Take your eyes off the monkey and you are likely to find yourself in trouble, so assume a relaxed urgency. Leave not so much as a crack in your defenses for the trickster to find a way in. From the beginning of step 1, use your head, neck, and eyes to maintain this focus. During step 3, relax deeply while sharpening your spirit and directing your attention forward. Imagine golden yellow light filling your body and radiating out and forward through your solar plexus.

LEFT SIDE

Now repeat the posture, but this time perform a mirror image of it, turning to the left instead of to the right.

2 Sit deeper into your right (back) leg and, keeping the weight forward, step back with your left foot. Rest it, toes first, a shoulder's width behind and left of your right foot, aligned east–west. Meanwhile, fold your right elbow, moving the hand palm down near your right ear, and drop your left arm, rolling it toward your body, palm facing. Your right fingers point to your left palm.

1 Keeping your weight mainly on your left (back) leg, turn your spine to the left. Let your right arm travel forward (west), palm down, drop your left arm, then arc it up and out to the side, to finish palm facing forward.

2 Keeping your weight seated in your front (left leg), step back with your right foot. Rest the toes a shoulder's width behind and right of the left foot, aligning the foot along the east–west axis. Meanwhile, fold the left elbow and move the hand palm down near the left ear; and dropping the right arm, roll it toward you, palm facing. The left fingers point to your right palm.

3 Transfer your weight to your back (right) foot, bringing your left toes round to face forward (west), and drop your left elbow so the palm faces forward opposite the left shoulder. The right hand falls, palm up, beside your right hip. Finish with 90% of your weight on your back (right) leg and 10% on your left leg, your feet parallel, a shoulder's width apart, facing west.

3 Transfer your weight to your back (left) foot, bringing your right toes round to face forward (west), and drop your right elbow, so your right palm faces west opposite your right shoulder. Your left hand falls, palm up, beside your left hip. Finish with 90% of your weight on your back (left) leg and 10% on your front (right) leg, your feet parallel, a shoulder width apart, facing west. Do not lock your front leg at the knee.

RIGHT SIDE

Perform the posture a third time, this time repeating the first position, turning to the right again.

1 **2** **3**

start position

DIAGONAL FLYING

Chen, thunder or arousing energy, is the trigram associated with Diagonal Flying, and it generates boldness. It is a celebration, an opportunity to shout fearlessly about the brilliance and passion of one's life. This posture is an embodiment of Split, one of the four secondary postures. It is the second posture to take place along the diagonal. At the beginning, the focus is on collecting the golden light that radiated out of the body at the end of the last sequence. At the finish, let the brilliant luminescence, now gathered up, burst into the body and be anchored there by the left hand, but fly out skyward through the right.

1 *From the start position, turn left as far as your hips allow. Meanwhile, your arms make a gathering movement, the left arm arching up to turn palm down opposite the center of your chest; the right hand dropping below the left to rest opposite the lower pelvis.*

VISUALIZATION

Begin step 1 by focusing on the yellow light still streaming from your solar plexus. Imagine gathering it up into a ball, and carrying it through step 2 until it reenters the body in the final movement. During step 3, notice split energy in the opposing nature of your rising right arm and dropping left one. Feel the anchoring energy of the left hand in contrast with the buoyant flight of the right arm. Feel full and radiant. As the movement ends you should feel entirely worthy of occupying the shape and space you are in.

2 *Relax your spine, which naturally turns to the right, and prepare to step by releasing all weight from your right foot. Lift your heel slightly, keeping the ball of your foot in contact with the ground. At this point you feel gathered, contained, and in transit.*

3 *Sitting deeply into your left leg, take a big step round with your right foot, placing it heel first toward the northeast.*

ARMS AND HANDS

As your weight moves to your right (front) leg during step 4, let your right arm fly upward, to extend palm up along the northeast diagonal. Look at the tip of your right middle finger, which is at eye level. Your left arm moves earthward toward your left thigh, palm down.

4 *Finish in a bow and arrow stance along the northeast diagonal, with 70% of your weight on your front (right) leg and 30% on your back leg, and your left foot aligned directly northward.*

start position

WAVING HANDS IN CLOUDS

The postures now leave the diagonal to align along the east–west axis. Waving Hands generates the energy of Ward Off, a primary movement. It moves from side to side – a sequence of energy-building side steps facing north is repeated on the right, then on the left. Repeatedly turning the spine massages the kidneys, and successively drawing up each hand promotes energy flow between the earthy vibrations of the root center and the finer ones of the heart, benefiting grounding and balance. Drawing energy from the solar plexus to the heart links celebrating personal power with achieving harmony with others.

POINTS TO WATCH

At the start, be aware of gathering in. At the end your hands hold a ball, a position that is repeated three times on the right side and three times on the left. Transferring weight from left to right coordinates with the arm movements, so be aware of the left arm floating up as you turn left, and vice versa; of the palms facing in the mid-position (see box); and when your weight is on the left and you face left, your left hand is on top of the ball, but when you face right and balance on the right, your right hand on top.

ADJUSTMENT STEP

Make a small step forward with the left foot to a position twice shoulder width from the right foot. Transfer your weight from right leg to left. This positions you for the next step. Finish with the left foot pointing north and the right foot northeast, heels aligned on the east–west axis.

1 RIGHT SIDE

Sit all your weight into your front (right) leg and, pivoting on the ball of your left foot, turn right (east). While turning, draw your right hand toward you and swivel the forearm, bringing the hand palm down opposite the center of your chest. Your left hand, palm upward, moves level with your lower pelvis. Your left leg rests behind, toes on the ground, heel lifted.

MID-POSITION

As the weight builds in your left leg and your spine turns left in steps 2, 4, and 6, allow your left hand to rise and your right hand to fall. As your body turns north, rotate your left palm to face your upper chest, and your right palm to face your lower

pelvis. From this mid-position, continue turning left while slowly rotating your left palm down and your right palm up.

While you turn in steps 3 and 5, your right hand rises and your left hand falls. As you face north in the mid-position, both palms turn to face your body.

4 LEFT SIDE

Sitting all your weight into your right leg and keeping the feet parallel, step west with the left foot, placing it twice shoulder width to the left of the right foot. Your left arm floats up, palm facing. Turn left as far as you can while dropping your right hand level with your lower pelvis and slowly turning the palm up. You finish holding a ball, left hand on top, palm down, right hand beneath, palm up; and with 60% of your weight on your left leg and 40% on your right leg.

5 RIGHT SIDE

Now repeat movement 3, Right Side, illustrated opposite.

2 LEFT SIDE

Turn left as far as you can, pointing your right foot north by pivoting on the heel. Finish with your feet parallel , 60% of your weight on your left leg, and 40% on your right leg.

3 RIGHT SIDE

Sit deeply into your left leg and place your right foot parallel to it one shoulder's width away. Draw your weight from left leg to right, imagining it traveling underground, while turning your spine to the right as far as your hips comfortably allow. Finish facing northeast.

6 LEFT SIDE

Repeat movement 4 Left Side, illustrated above, before proceeding to the first movement of Single Whip on the next page.

start position

SINGLE WHIP

Here, Single Whip reappears to mark a change in direction and momentum after the sequence ended by Waving Hands. In its third appearance, this posture has a new, enjoyable role: to develop flowing coordination. It is energized by the ball of energy caught between the hands at the end of Waving Hands. Its slow unfolding introduces a change, ready for the next part of the form. Enjoy the sweeping arm and hand movements of step 1. Take the longest possible step into the bow and arrow stance, since it boosts the circulation.

1 Step directly northward with your right leg and transfer all your weight to it while turning your spine to the northeast. As you finish, your left foot rests behind, heel lifted.

2 Relax and turn your spine left, pivoting on the ball of your left foot. With all the balance in your right leg, take a long step west with your left foot, into a bow and arrow stance. The left palm turns to face the left shoulder.

3 Transfer your weight to the left (front) leg, imagining the weight travelling underground. Straighten your back leg and turn your hips to the west. The toes of the back foot turn to an angle of 45° while turning your left palm to face away opposite your shoulder. Finish with 70% of your weight on your front leg and 30% on the back leg.

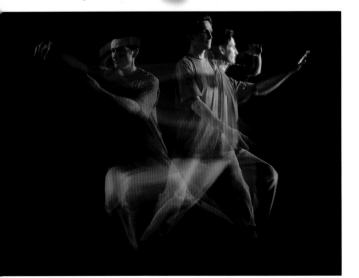

SWOOPING HAND

As you transfer your weight from your left (back) leg in step 1, you drop your right hand, forming it into a hook before raising and extending it along the diagonal (northeast). Meanwhile, your left hand drops and swoops up, rotating to turn the palm up in a supporting role opposite your solar plexus. You maintain the hook hand through the next posture, Squatting Single Whip, and only release it at the beginning of Golden Rooster on page 118.

SQUATTING SINGLE WHIP

Single Whip is followed by a variation on itself, Squatting Single Whip. Elegant and aesthetically pleasing, this is a strong, dynamic posture and a great favorite. It refreshes the body, opens the hips and pelvis, and massages the colon. It exercises the legs, boosting blood circulation and cleansing the lymph fluid that bathes the tissues. This posture is strongly cyclical – feel the drawing back in step 1 as the first quadrant of a circle, followed by moving down, forward, and up. The right hand remains in a hook shape throughout the posture.

1 *Turn your right toes to the rear diagonal (northeast) and your left palm toward the center of your chest. At the same time, bring your weight back to your right leg.*

2 *Folding in the hips, drop your spine vertically as if you were squatting through your right leg, aligning your knees with your feet. Keep most of your weight back while connecting your front foot with the ground. Let your front (left) leg bend. Drop your left hand, pointing your fingers to the earth.*

3 *Turn your left toes out to the southwest, turn your hips to face west and rotate your left palm outward (facing north). Continue to drop vertically.*

4 *Bring your weight forward, while lifting your left hand to rest palm down outside and beside your left thigh. Your right hook hand remains out to the side. Your weight is mainly in your left (front) leg, the toes pointing southwest. The right toes point northwest.*

VISUALIZATION

Squatting Single Whip is also aptly called Snake Creeps Down – during step 2, visualize yourself filling with a cascade of cosmic energy which descends from the top of your head to the base of your spine as your left hand pulls it down through your body, allowing it to earth. Imagine this force as powerfully cleansing and allow it to inspire you.

start position

GOLDEN ROOSTER STANDS ON ONE LEG

The fact that the golden rooster is standing on one leg indicates its role: to train the balance and develop poise. This posture is therefore performed first on the right side and then on the left. It takes movements begun earlier and carries them on. Its first step doubles as the last step of Squatting Single Whip on page 117; and the hook hand created at the start of Single Whip on page 116 is now released as if throwing the explosive ball carried from Waving Hands on page 115 to the ground. The explosion bounces back through the right-hand fingers and returns to the sky.

RIGHT SIDE

1 *Sitting your weight into your left leg, sweep your right arm downward, releasing the hook hand. Point the fingers earthward.*

POINTS TO WATCH

Work on deepening your consciousness of your sense of balance. Imagine your body aligns with a pillar rising through the foot which supports your balance, and through your hip to the top of your head. Although you are standing, see yourself sitting on your hip, which is solidly earthed through your foot. Through the posture, maintain a keen awareness of the polarity between the energy dropping through the earthed leg and the skyward energy of your raised arm and hand.

2 *Continue the arm sweep upward while lifting your right leg. Finish standing on your left leg, your right thigh parallel to the ground, the toes pointing down. Your hips and right thigh face west, your left hand has risen slightly to hip level, palm turned down, and your right-hand fingers point skyward.*

LEFT SIDE

1 *Keeping your weight on your left leg, step down and back with your right foot, resting it half a shoulder width from your left foot and a shoulder width behind it, the toes facing northwest. Lower your right hand level with your right hip, palm turned down. Your hips face west. Feel the coordination between the foot on the ground and the palm of the hand earthing.*

2 *Drop naturally into balancing on your right leg and point the left toes west.*

3 *Release your left hand and leg so they move up. Your hips and thigh face west, the thigh parallel with the ground and the toes pointing down. Your left-hand fingers finish pointing up, and the right hand at hip level and facing down.*

STATIC STANDING

Many beginners have poor balance and those who find this posture difficult may benefit from practicing the second part of step 1 as a static posture, starting by standing for perhaps half a minute on each leg in turn and working up to five minutes. You may need to begin by keeping the toes in contact with the ground and lifting just the heel, gradually working up to holding the thigh parallel with the ground and keeping it there for longer and longer periods.

VARIATION ON A ROOSTER THEME

To create a more dynamic posture, repeat step 2, right side, but sit deeper into your right leg, and bring your left knee up to touch your left elbow. Then repeat step 3, left side, bringing your right knee up to touch your right elbow.

start position

SEPARATE RIGHT FOOT

This posture continues the role of Golden Rooster in developing balance, but takes it further. In the last posture both legs were static during the balancing, in Separate Right Foot the body balances on the left leg and the feet are separated during a wide, swinging kick with the right foot. This movement is balanced by repeating the posture on the left side. The posture makes a dynamic link between sky and earth and the polarity of outward and inward. Beginning with pull in from the sky down to the earth below the feet.

1 *Keeping most of your weight on the front (right) leg, step back with your left foot and place it facing southwest. Meanwhile, turn to the front right diagonal as if catching something between your arms. Look along the diagonal, gazing upward slightly.*

CROSSING HANDS

As you move one foot next to the other during step 2, make a full circle with your arms, finishing with the hands crossed, right hand on the outside, opposite your throat. In Separate Left Foot cross your left hand over your right hand. Direct your awareness clearly inward and feel your alignment into the earth.

HANDS AND ARMS

Just before you kick in step 3, open your arms, turning the palms out. In Separate Right Foot align the right arm with the right leg just above shoulder height, extending the left arm out to the side for balance. In Separate Left Foot align your left arm with your left leg and extend your right arm out to the side.

2 *Moving your weight to your back (left) leg, pull down with your arms.*

3 *Turn your spine as far left as you can, so you face southwest. Keeping all your weight on the left leg, rest your right foot, heel lifted, beside the left.*

4 *Balancing on the left leg, turn your hips to face west and your head northwest, and release your right foot in a swinging kick along the northwest diagonal. Do not point the toes up. Your leg remains lifted, thigh parallel to the floor, knee bent, toes pointing down.*

VISUALIZATION

In step 1, direct your awareness along the diagonal and extend it out and up as if forging a link with the sky. In step 2, imagine yourself pulling something down from the sky which passes through your feet into the center of the earth. Feel a surge of energy rise from the earth's center during step 4. Surf this with your mind and let it flood your body, so the kick you make at the end of the posture comes from deep within, and your mind moves clearly outward to accompany the move.

SEPARATE LEFT FOOT

O nce the right foot is extended in the kick, allow the leg to fold at the knee and the lower leg to rest, and then turn to the left diagonal to repeat the posture on the left side. While aligning with the left diagonal, accompany the movement of your "catching" arms by focusing your awareness to the southwest. Begin this movement with the same pulling down motion as in Separate Right Foot, but after that, all movements are reversed. The constant movements of this posture stimulate circulation and increase mental dexterity, with a shifting of awareness inward and then outward.

1 *To align with the diagonal, turn your hips southwest, step back (northeast) with the right foot and keeping your weight forward, point it northwest. As if to catch something while turning, move your right hand opposite the left elbow and extend your left arm along the southwest diagonal.*

2 *Move your weight to your back (right) leg while pulling down with your arms.*

3 *Turn your spine to the right and rest your left foot next to your right foot, heel lifted slightly. Circling your arms, finish in the crossing hands position facing northwest, your weight on the right leg.*

4 *Balancing on the right leg, turn your hips to the west, open your arms, turning the palms out, and kick with your left foot along the southwest diagonal, keeping your toes pointing forward.*

"CATCHING" ARMS

As you turn to the diagonal in step 1, drop your left arm to rest opposite your right elbow, turning the palm up. Raise your right hand, turning the palm down and extending the arm along the diagonal. Finish with arms and hands positioned as if to catch something between them as you turn.

start position

BRUSH KNEE AND PUSH

It is in the seven postures illustrated on the following six pages that the form of Dr. Chi Chiang-tao differs from the original 37-Step Short Form created by his master, Cheng Man-ch'ing (see pages 84–5). Anyone already familiar with the original version is invited to try out this variation on the Cheng Man-ch'ing form. For those who prefer to continue practicing what they have learned, the original is illustrated on page 85. The variation begins with Brush Knee and Push. This posture also appears on pages 99 and 101, but there it begins in a slightly different way. In this position in the form it acts as a breather.

1 *Turn your hips as far as you can to the right and soften your right palm by relaxing the hand with the palm open and facing forward. Fold your left elbow to bring your left hand in.*

2 *Step with your left foot into a bow and arrow stance to finish facing west, moving 70% of your weight to your front leg.*

NEEDLES AT SEA BOTTOM

Feel the arm movements in step 2 as a drawing in, and those in step 3 as a sending out. Enjoy the strong downward momentum of the pull, which begins in step 3 when you direct your mental awareness diagonally downward, and uses the whole body. Needles at Sea Bottom massages the colon, which stimulates it to function more efficiently.

HANDS

Emphasizing the downward momentum of step 4, your hands also drop automatically. Rest your left palm on your right hand to support it as it pulls down. The fingers of your right hand finish pointing directly to the earth.

1 *Step with your right foot to rest it just behind the left, while transferring your weight to the left leg. Direct your mind out and forward to focus it on what you are going to do next.*

2 *Move your weight to the right (rear) leg, turn a little to the right, and bring your left palm next to your right elbow.*

3 *Release your left foot and place it in a cat stance. Straighten your hips toward the front (west), send your right hand down diagonally away from you, and slide your left palm down onto your right wrist.*

4 *Keeping 90% of your weight seated in your right leg, fold in your hips by bending your knees and inclining your spine forward. Keep your spine aligned from the coccyx to the head.*

IRON FAN

This is a strong posture that grows as if from a planted seed. Like a tree it has a rising momentum in the form of a trunk and a spreading, branchlike shape. It imparts strength, focus, and warrior energy which can benefit women as well as men. As you follow step 2, let the energy of the developing posture fill your body and extend along your spreading arms. As you deepen your stance, the spread of your arms extends. Anchored firmly by your legs, your eyes focused to the right of your left hand on the space where your right-hand fingers are projecting, allow the warrior in your soul to flood your body.

2 *Bend your right knee, drop to the right, and make a wide step forward with the left foot into a bow and arrow stance, facing west.*

3 *Move your weight forward, resting 70% on the front leg, turn right so your hips face northwest, and turn your right foot out through 90° to point north.*

1 *Keeping your weight in the right leg, draw upright from the hips, and the left leg lifts. Align the thigh parallel to the ground. Let your elbows drop and the hands float and rest, quietly alert, in front of the body. Maintain internal equilibrium while feeling the posture's upward growth.*

ARMS AND HANDS

During step 2, extend your left arm forward and slowly spread your arms out. Move the hand well back to open the palm fully toward the right (northwest) diagonal. Keep the elbow down.
During step 3 draw your right hand back, rotating the forearm outward and bringing it parallel to the ground. Your right hand finishes beside your face, palm facing out and fingers facing west.

start position

TURN BODY, CHOP AND PUSH

These movements take the warrior energy from Iron Fan into action, and in a coordinated dance between hands and feet express the energy of the cosmos and the earth. They bring a sense of passion. The fist you make with your right hand draws power from the earth, while your left hand draws energy from the sky, and the two fuel the forward-moving fist and the push at the finish. The posture teaches coordination between stepping, weight shifts, hands, and feet. Its intricate movements might seem awkward and difficult at first, but try to feel the momentum created by turning the spine and moving the weight.

2 *Keep turning right to face northeast and move most of your weight back to the left leg. Lift the right heel and pivot on the ball of the foot. Unfold your elbow and drop the fist, resting it outside and next to your right thigh.*

HANDS AND ARMS

As you turn in step 1, bring your left hand above your head, palm away. Lower your right forearm to chest level, making a fist of the right hand, facing down.

1 *Turn to the right (north) as far as your hips allow, bringing most of your weight into your right leg. Follow it with your left foot, which pivots on the heel to finish pointing north.*

3 *Step forward (east) with your right foot into a bow and arrow stance, softening your right elbow and circling the fist up and forward, the back of the hand opposite your right shoulder. Meanwhile, lower the left hand, resting it palm facing close to your right elbow. Your feet make a 90° angle, a shoulder's width apart, most weight on the back leg.*

VISUALIZATION

Focus the turn in step 1 into your right elbow, and on a line running from left fingers down to right fist. In step 2, direct your spirit into the space you turn toward. Feel the balance on your left side and the power of the open shape made by your left hand connecting with the sky and the anchoring right fist. In step 3 focus on coordinating three moves. Imagine your left hand pulling down cosmic energy as you step. Direct your mind forward in step 4, drawing power through your left arm.

4 *Move 70% of your weight forward to your front leg, and turn your left toes northeast. Simultaneously withdraw your right fist to rest it next to your right hip, turn to the front, and push from your back leg to give a forward push with your left palm.*

BRING DOWN

This move links Turn Body, Chop and Push with Punch and has a strong grounding effect. Begin by reaching up with your right hand in one large rolling movement. The bringing down is expressed as the right hand falls. End by storing energy in the hui yin energy center in the lower pelvis.

1 *Keep your weight on your front leg, open your right hip and turn left slightly to face north. Simultaneously release your fist and send your right hand up to shoulder level, palm facing left and fingers pointing forward.*

2 *Move most of your weight to the back (left) leg.*

HANDS

As your weight moves left, drop your left hand, rolling the palm up, and drop your right hand, turning the palm down. Finish with your left palm turned up beside your left hip and your right palm turned down in front of and crossing the path of your left hand, making a T shape.

PUNCH (2)

Here, the movement blends into a repeat of Punch. First make the adjustment move, then follow steps 3, 4, 5 and 6 from Punch on pages 102–03. Concentrate on focusing the root energy you have drawn from your pelvis, and put your whole being, body and soul, into the punch.

ADJUSTMENT MOVE

Release your right foot to step, make a fist with your right hand, and turn to the right to finish facing southeast. Accompany the turn with a sweeping movement of your right, fist arm. Now move directly into step 3 of Punch on page 102, and follow with steps 4–6 on page 103. This adjustment move is equivalent to steps 1 and 2 of Punch on page 102–3. From it, move smoothly into steps 3–6 shown here. The arm movements are exactly the same as in steps 3–6 of Punch on pages 102–3.

4 + 5   **3**   **2**   **1**

start position

KICK WITH HEEL

This first posture might still more descriptively be called "Embrace Emptiness, Cross Hands, and Kick With Heel." A phase of emptiness occurs at the beginning of Kick With Heel, following the fullness of the energy held after the punch that ends the previous posture. As you begin, experience total emptiness. Step 2 returns you to a fullness rooted in the earth's center. The right heel kick comes at the end from an inward gathering, centering and focusing. Kick with Heel improves coordination between mind and body.

POINTS TO WATCH

From inside the full shape created in step 2 by your crossed hands, feel the kick emerge during step 3. Do not hold onto it but allow it to travel fully out, imagining that you release it along the southeast diagonal. You kick with the heel of the right foot, unlike the kick in Separate Feet on pages 120–21, which is more of a toe kick. In this posture the leg swings higher, stretching the back of the leg. Try not to kick too high or with too much force. Use the momentum you build up to glide the leg smoothly forward.

1 *Release the right fist you formed in the last posture, and drop both elbows, keeping the palms facing up at a natural angle of about 45° from the horizontal. Now, with your weight almost entirely in your back (right) leg and the left toes lifted, turn to the northeast diagonal.*

2 *Sit into your front (left) leg, move all your weight forward, and cross your right arm over your left in front of your body, your wrists crossing opposite your throat. Your right leg rests behind, heel lifted.*

3 *Open your arms up and out, turning the palms outward and pointing your right arm southeast. At the same time send your right leg in a swinging kick northeast along the diagonal, the heel pushing forward strongly.*

4 *After the kick, allow your leg while still in the air to bend and relax at the knee, and the foot to rest, pointing downward.*

BRUSH RIGHT KNEE AND PUSH

Kick With Heel is followed by Brush Right Knee and Push, here in its role as a breather between two sequences of postures. Its fourth appearance in the form mirrors the version on page 122 exactly. Remember to be aware of the drawing-in momentum of the first part of the posture, and the sending-out feeling during the second.

1 *Keeping your balance on the left leg, turn left until your hips face northeast, folding your right arm and softening your left palm so it faces forward. Your right hand comes to rest palm down opposite the center of your chest.*

2 *Step with your right foot to lead into a right bow and arrow stance facing directly east and with 70% of your weight in your front (right) foot and 30% on your back leg.*

REFERENCE GUIDE

- The action of sitting the weight into a leg is described on pages 68–9.
- The bow and arrow stance referred to in Brush Right Knee and Push is illustrated on page 71.

start position

BRUSH LEFT KNEE AND PUNCH DOWNWARD

At this point, where the Cheng Man-ch'ing variation and the Chi Chiang-tao versions of the form rejoin, postures from earlier in the form reappear, marking the beginning of a change. First, the Brush Knee posture is expressed again, but this time as a punch instead of a push. Brush Left Knee And Punch Downward develops a sense of solid strength. It can transform the energy of indecision into direction.

1 *Turn right to the southeast diagonal, anchor on your rear leg and place your right foot on the diagonal. Drop your left hand as the weight moves back.*

2 *Sit your weight into your right leg and rest your left foot behind, heel lifted. Form a fist with your left hand as the weight moves into the front leg.*

3 *Step east with your left foot and transfer your weight forward, forming a a bow and arrow stance.*

4 *As your weight moves, the downward-facing palm of your moving left hand clears your left knee to finish forward. Powered by your straightening back leg, punch down, then along. Finish facing east with your spine inclined and 80% of your weight on your front (left) leg and 20% on your back leg.*

VISUALIZATION

Feel the link between the sinking of the body and the floating of the arms. Imagine the incoming energy as a sign of your inner change from uncertainty to commitment, and capture it with your moving left hand. In step 4 you transform it into the solid, committed punch.

WARD OFF RIGHT

This posture is a repeat of Ward Off Right on page 90, but it originates at a different point. Where the first Ward Off Right grew out of a contained solidity, this one comes directly from a solid commitment. While bringing your weight forward during step 2, feel the wave of Ward Off energy passing up through and in front of your body and raising sexual energy from the hui yin center in the lower pelvis to the throat. Ward Off Right moves into Rollback, then Press, Push, and Single Whip, marking the end of the second sequence of postures.

1 *Turn to the left and place your foot on the diagonal. Release the fist and draw your right hand back and in with a sense of gathering and raising. Your left fingers and hips point northeast.*

2 *Drop your weight onto your front (left) leg and lift your right heel, while moving your right hand up and forward.*

3 *Step with your right foot into a bow and arrow stance facing east. Your right hand rests, palm facing, at throat level; the left fingers point to the right palm. Your weight finishes 70% on the front leg, 30% on the back leg.*

ROLLBACK

The energy raised in Ward Off Right is again absorbed and earthed by this repeat of Rollback on page 91.

PRESS

Now move smoothly into Press, following the same sequence of movements shown on page 92.

PUSH

From Press, progress without a break into Push, as shown on page 92.

SINGLE WHIP

This sequence of repeated postures ends with the now familiar Single Whip, following the steps on pages 94–5.

太 129 極

start position

FAIR LADY WEAVES THE SHUTTLE I

This posture has four positions which repeat, two on the left and two on the right. The first is illustrated here and the second, third and fourth on the following pages. Each non-cardinal direction is visited in counterclockwise order – northeast, northwest, southwest, and southeast – against which the body weaves a web of movements in a delightful play. A complete circle is covered in the Fair Lady sequence of postures.

1 *Sit into your right leg and turn to the right. Your left foot turns north. Soften your left arm, drop the elbow slightly, and turn your left palm to face the center of your chest. Your right hand forms a hook shape. Concentrate on a sense of gathering in through the first steps of this posture.*

2 *Simultaneously release your right hook hand, bring your weight onto the left leg, and continue turning right, lifting the right foot and placing it facing east. Draw in your left arm palm up until the fingers are near your right elbow. The right arm is relaxed, palm away, opposite your shoulder.*

POINTS TO WATCH

Sending out is followed by gathering in, so the atmosphere changes as the movements progress. One effect of this can be to open the consciousness. When the weight changes, the hands change: this recurrent pattern is especially clear in the Fair Lady postures, so watch for places where the weight moves. In steps 2 and 3 take as large a step as you can, since this aids flexibility and mobility, especially in the hip joints.

HANDS STEP 3

When the weight changes, the hands change. As your weight shifts onto your right leg in step 3, relax your arms and move your right hand down past the front of your left palm, which is rising to face your throat. Finish with the fingers of your right hand pointing toward your left palm. Notice how the right hand draws something down and in, the left hand draws something up.

3 *Slowly move all your weight onto your right leg, following the eastward direction of your right foot. Your left leg rests behind, heel lifted.*

4 *Without moving your arms, release your left foot to step into a bow and arrow stance along the northeast diagonal.*

5 *Bring 70% of your weight forward to your front foot. Feel the carefully gathered energy transform into a bold outward expression.*

HANDS STEP 5

As your weight moves forward to your left leg in step 5, your left arm moves up and rolls palm outward, turning to the sky. Your right hand, quietly tucked in behind the left, appears and pushes boldly forward. Notice the link between the left hand meeting the sky and the right hand sending outward. Nurture this connection.

start position

FAIR LADY WEAVES THE SHUTTLE 2

The first position in the Fair Lady sequence of postures (see pages 130–31) moves without a break into the second position, below. The cycle finishes with Ward Off Left on the following pages. The Fair Lady links the crown energy center to the heart center, encouraging communion with the surrounding space. Practiced outdoors, these postures encourage communication with nature. Indoors, they might clear space or the atmosphere in a room or in a new house.

POINTS TO WATCH

Here, you make a large, sweeping turn around 270° to finish facing northwest. Be aware of the difference between the outward expression at the end of Fair Lady 1 on page 130 and the gathering movements here. Notice how your hands weave, the right hand coming in and down before pulling up and out, the left coming toward, then down. Remember: when the weight changes, the hands change.

1 Move your weight to the right leg, and pivoting on the left heel, turn the left foot 90°. Rotating the hips southeast, roll your left arm down and toward you so the palm faces your throat, and roll your right hand toward the solar plexus, turning up the palm.

2 Bring all your weight onto your back leg while turning right, lifting the right heel to adjust the foot's position. Move the right foot about 9 inches to the right and place it on the ground facing south.

3 Move your weight to the right leg, lift your left heel, and pivot on the ball of your left foot until your hips face southwest. The right foot points south and the left rests behind, heel lifted, aligned on the diagonal.

4 Move your weight back to your left foot which, with your hips, faces southwest. Slide your right foot toward it. Turning your spine to the right, move your right foot back past the left foot along the northwest diagonal, placing it heel first, toes pointing northwest. Your hips face west.

5 Bring 70% of your weight to the right leg, turn your hips northwest, and your left toes west, finishing in a bow and arrow stance along the northwest diagonal. Roll your right arm above your head, turning the palm north; the left hand pushes forward opposite the shoulder along the diagonal.

CHANGING HANDS

As your weight moves back in step 2 of Fair Lady 2 and 4, roll your left hand, palm toward the right, and rest it opposite your solar plexus, palm away. Drop your right elbow and float the right hand up, passing the descending left palm, to rest it opposite the center of your chest. Your left fingers point to the right palm and remain there during steps 3 and 4.

FAIR LADY WEAVES THE SHUTTLE 3

In this, the third position in the cycle, the moves join in the counterclockwise pattern being woven.

1 *Bring your weight to your back leg while rolling your left palm to face your solar plexus. Drop your right elbow, bringing your right arm to face palm away opposite your right shoulder. Release your right foot to place it pointing west, keeping your weight back.*

2 *Transfer your weight to your right leg, raising your left hand to face your throat. The right arm drops and faces palm away, and the fingers point at the left palm.*

3 *Step with your left foot into a bow and arrow stance along the southwest diagonal. As your weight moves to your left leg, raise your left arm and roll the palm out and up. Your right hand pushes forward. Notice the link between the left hand meeting the sky and the right hand sending outward.*

FAIR LADY WEAVES THE SHUTTLE 4

The movements are almost identical to those in Fair Lady 2, but this position starts in the southwest and finishes facing southeast to complete the four non-cardinal directions.

1 *Move your weight to your right leg, then pivoting on your left heel turn the foot 90° to point north-west, and turn your hips north-west. As you turn, roll your left arm down toward your throat, and your right hand toward your solar plexus, palm up.*

2 *Bring all your weight to your back leg while turning right, lifting the right heel to adjust the foot. Meanwhile, your hands change as shown in the box (opposite). Move the right foot about 9 inches to the right and place it facing north.*

3 *Transfer your weight to your right leg, lift the left heel, and turning the hips northeast, pivot on your left foot. Your right foot, points north, your left foot resting behind it, heel lifted, aligned along the northeast–southwest diagonal.*

4 *Move your weight back to your left foot, which, with your hips, faces northeast. Slide your right foot toward it. Turning your spine right, move your right foot back past the left foot along the diagonal, placing it heel first, facing southeast. Your hips face east.*

5 *Bring 70% of your weight to the right leg, turning your hips southeast and your left toes to the east, adopting a bow and arrow stance along the southeast diagonal. Simultaneously roll your left arm down toward your throat, and your right hand toward your solar plexus, turning the palm up. Roll your right arm above the head, turning the palm southward; and push your left hand forward opposite the left shoulder.*

start position

WARD OFF LEFT

The moves on these two pages mark the end of the Fair Lady sequence of postures and the start of a series of postures that ends the form. Ward Off Left ends as on page 89, but its beginning is different. It emerges from the movements woven through the four positions of Fair Lady on the preceding pages, and although it concentrates on gathering in, it has a different feeling. It delivers a sense of containment and completion. From Ward Off Left the sequence merges into Ward Off Right, Rollback, Press, and Push, and ends with Single Whip, all played out exactly as on pages 89–93.

1 *Keeping your weight on your front leg, draw the right foot round to point east. Drop the left hand and roll it palm up to rest opposite the lower pelvis; and rest the right hand palm down opposite the center of your chest. At the end, your hands hold a ball.*

2 *Step north with your left leg in preparation for a bow and arrow stance, placing the heel down first. Your feet make a 90° angle, a shoulder's width apart and about twice this distance front to back. Do not lock your left leg at the knee.*

3 *Transfer your weight forward, while raising the left arm and lowering the right hand. Pushing down with your back foot straightens your back leg, turns your body north, and turns the toes of the back foot 45° to face northeast. Finish with 70% of your weight on the back leg and 30% on the front.*

VISUALIZATION

The sense of gathering in step 1 comes from the magic woven by the Fair Lady postures. Imagine holding the Earth in your hands, and in step 2, filling with the energy of the primary posture Ward Off, which comes from holding the world. Note how the posture's final shape feels contained, and the right hand acts as an anchor into the earth.

ARMS

From step 2, your arms continue moving slowly, so that by step 3 your left arm is opposite the center of your chest, comfortably curved and with the palm facing, and your right hand is opposite your left thigh with either the fingers or the palm facing earthward.

WARD OFF RIGHT

This repeat of the posture shown on page 90 energizes the whole body by drawing the creative sexual energy of Ward Off through it.

ROLLBACK

Here, Rollback appears in the form for the fourth time. From Ward Off Right, turn your awareness to the southeast-northwest diagonal, and follow the same steps as on page 91.

PRESS

The sequence now glides into Press. Follow the same movements as on page 92.

PUSH

Press moves without interruption into Push, where energy is once again gathered in, as shown on page 93.

SINGLE WHIP

Single Whip marks the end of the sequence and the start of a new one. Follow the steps shown on pages 94–5.

start position

SQUATTING SINGLE WHIP

In its second appearance in the form Squatting Single Whip (also called Snake Creeps Down) brings cosmic energy from the sky to earth through the body. At the end it merges into a new posture with a strong, warrior-like position, called Step Forward to the Seven Stars, perhaps a reference to a constellation – the Big Dipper or Plough which has seven stars. These postures work together, so the energy of Squatting Single Whip fills the Seven Stars.

2 *Folding in your hips and keeping your knees and feet aligned, drop your spine vertically as if you were squatting through your right leg. Keep your weight back on your right leg, your front foot connected with the ground, and the knee bent.*

3 *Turn your left toes to the southwest, and rotate the left palm to face north.*

1 *Keeping the right hand in a hook shape, bring your weight back to your right leg while turning your right toes to the northeast diagonal. Move your left palm toward the center of your chest.*

STEP FORWARD TO THE SEVEN STARS

start position

The position of the body in this posture resembles the Plough constellation, with the right foot, knee and hip, and the two elbows and fists forming a similar pattern whose attributes are strength, focus, and integrity. Begin the posture with your right hand still in a hook shape, out to the side.

3 *Circle your right arm up forming a fist, and cross the right wrist over the left, the wrists sticking. Meanwhile, step forward (west), placing the right foot in a cat stance. Your balance runs down your left side, with 90% of your weight on the back leg and 10% on the right leg.*

2 *Release the hook hand as you sweep your right arm down.*

1 *Bringing the weight forward, circle the left hand up and forward, making a fist and resting it 12 inches from your chin, the back of the hand facing up. Most of your weight is on the front foot which points southwest. The right toes point northwest.*

STEP BACK TO RIDE TIGER

The role of this posture is to ready the player to meet any adversary that may appear. The warrior of the last position deals in an open and impartial manner with the need of the moment, defusing and earthing the ferocious, threatening tiger energy.

1 *Release your fists, dropping your hands as you step back with your right foot and point the toes southwest, but keep your weight forward on the left leg.*

2 *Move your weight back, and your left foot toward your body, and, keeping the ball of the foot in contact with the ground, adopt a cat stance. Meanwhile, circle the right hand to face palm forward level with and to the right of your face. Soften and open your face. Move your left hand across your left thigh, the palm facing down.*

TAI CHI TERMS

Stick: to keep two parts of the body (or two tai chi players) close together even while moving.

VISUALIZATION

As both hands drop downward and you step back, focus on earthing, emptying, and neutralizing a difficult incoming force. In the final position, feel your open, balanced state of mind and body as a place from which wise choices can be made.

start position

TURN AND SWEEP LOTUS

Turn and Sweep Lotus, with its swirling movement and explosive sweep-kick at the end, is like shouting an enjoyable "Hey!" in celebration of the form. The speed of the sweep brings a relief from the steady rhythm of the other postures. The turn in this posture can be difficult. It works well when the mind and body form a downward, inward spiral, but if it is perceived as a stressful movement, the body tenses up, upsetting the balance. This posture therefore improves balance and encourages good coordination.

1 *Keeping all your weight on your right leg, turn your hips and spine a little to the left, your left leg traveling with them. Meanwhile, begin to drop your right hand across your body to the level of your pelvis.*

VISUALIZATION

Learning how to break the pattern of "challenge equals stress" involves understanding how to drop the center of gravity in a challenging situation. The secret is to direct the attention inward at the beginning of the posture, and to visualize the center of gravity spiraling downward through the spinning right foot, and becoming a smooth pirouette with the transfer of weight to the left foot.

TURN AND SWEEP LOTUS

Imagine the turn in step 2 giving you a firmly grounded center of gravity, which drops through your spinning right foot and so into the earth. Let the sweeping kick in steps 5, 6, and 7 unfold from the internal focus of your attention in an expression of playfulness. Enjoy it and return to a poised state, centering your internal balance through your left leg.

2 *Lead with your left foot into a swirling 360° body turn to the right, pivoting on the ball of your right foot.*

3 *Halfway through the turn, place your left heel behind and left of your starting point, the toes pointing southwest. Meanwhile, turn your left palm to face forward. Your right hand rests level with the lower tantien.*

THE KICK

As it passes under your hands during the kick in step 6, let your right foot clip the fingers of both hands with a smacking sound. In order to make contact between foot and hand, you need to mobilize your hips and keep your knee high. This might take some practice, and if you find it impossible at first, concentrate on lifting your knee as high as you can without losing your balance.

4 *As your left foot touches down, your weight spirals through it into the ground. Continue pivoting on the ball of your right foot. As the turn ends, raise both arms. Finish with the hands, palm down, opposite the shoulder.*

5 *Anchor firmly in your left leg and lift your right knee, moving it left.*

6 *Sweep your right leg to the right across your body in a downward-curving arc.*

7 *Concentrate on lifting your knee as high as you can during the kick, without losing your balance.*

8 *Bring your leg back to the center and rest it, knee lifted and foot pointing down. The arms remain comfortably extended. Finish with your left foot pointing southwest and your body facing west.*

start position

BEND BOW TO SHOOT TIGER

Bend Bow to Shoot Tiger is the final posture in the form with a warrior stance and calls for disciplined movements and steady rhythm. It has a strong downward momentum and it restores a deep connection with the earth, from which comes the warrior stance at the end. It has a strong grounding effect and, like the Seven Stars on page 136, can give a feeling of strength, focus, and integrity. Maintaining the martial image, the posture moves into Punch, which has the same slow, even tempo. It is important by this stage of practice to try to relax the mind in order to achieve a smooth flow in the movements.

VISUALIZATION

Join the downward momentum of step 1 with your eyes, focusing on the earthing effect of this part of the move. Keep your spirit lifted. During step 2 your hands form fists softly but definitely, as if drawing on the energy of the earth. Feel the distance between the fists increase as the movement progresses, as if you were stretching a bow, and how the left fist in particular extends away from your strongly anchored body.

1 *Drop your spine and arms as you turn to the right, placing the right foot on the northwest diagonal. Your arms sweep down, palms facing down as if they were bringing something to earth. The left leg bends at the knee to allow the spine to drop. Keep your weight mainly on the back leg.*

2 *Continue to turn right as you form fists with both hands and circle them forward and up. The left foot points southwest; the right foot is a shoulder's width from it and forward in a stance to the northwest. Start to bring your weight forward, your fists rising.*

HANDS

Move 70% of your weight well forward to your front (right) foot during step 2, while raising your right fist level with the top of your head. Continue sending your left fist forward to finish comfortably opposite your solar plexus. If you were holding a pencil in your left hand, it would lean at an angle of 45° to the perpendicular.

PUNCH (3)

This posture first appeared on pages 102–03, but it emerges from a different place, so the movements in the first two steps are different. Releasing the left fist in step 1 gives a sense of letting go of Bend Bow To Shoot Tiger. The downward movement gives the impression of storing, as if you were gathering the warrior energy encountered through the form. From step 3 follow the movements shown on page 103, putting heart and soul into the punch in step 6.

1 *Sit into your right leg and release your left fist.*

2 *Step back with your left foot, and bringing your weight back, turn to the left. Rotate your left hand palm up while dropping it to rest beside your left thigh, and tilt your right fist (palm down, were it open) in front of your left fingers. Pivot on the ball of your right foot to face southwest.*

3 *From step 2, move into step 3 of the version of Punch on page 102, and continue through to step 6.*

HAND AND FIST

From the beginning of the turn in step 2, sweep your right fist, hand upward, in an arc to drop down by your right hip. Raise your left hand to coordinate with it, so that as your hip drops, your left hand faces – palm forward – the right front (northwest) diagonal. Your right hand, if you opened your fist, would face palm up. Follow this direction with your face and eyes.

start position

WITHDRAW AND PUSH

Two postures from early on – Withdraw and Push and Crossing Hands – recur, but although the same movements are repeated in the same order, there is a difference. The story woven by these two postures differs slightly from the tale they told earlier on in the form, because here they are concerned with its conclusion. They deliver a sense of integrating and calling together of all the moves in the form. Start by following the steps for Withdraw and Push on page 104.

VISUALIZATION

Compare the feeling of your open, empty hand with your closed fist and imagine dandelion seeds blown from your hand by the wind, or some other image that carries a sense of release, such as a white dove flying from your fingers. As you withdraw, maintain a sense that you are clearing the space of the story of the form. And as you push, see the movement as a wish to fill your life with clear, positive energy.

1 *Gently releasing the fist you formed in the last posture, move into the first step of Withdraw and Push, then follow steps 2 and 3.*

CROSSING HANDS

This final posture restores equilibrium. Follow the steps shown in Crossing Hands on page 105, concentrating on the strong, contained shape your body makes and its alignment, anchored in the earth and lifted to the sky. Open up to the universe before creating the final seal as your wrists cross.

COMPLETION

So much energy is held in the final moment. Like the last note in an opera, the sound and the energy of the form need to remain clear and linger after the movements are completed, leaving a sustained note of beauty and dignity. This moment deserves to be savored so that the energy so carefully built up through each posture is not lost but stored and nurtured. The form should create a rich treasury of energy on which body and soul can feed.

As your hands come down, feel this as a final clearing of the form and of your space. Finish with an acknowledgment of the reality of your situation: you are simply a human standing on the earth.

VISUALIZATION

Keep your awareness clearly focused on the final moves until the last one is made, then, after movement has ceased, pause for a moment of stillness. Taking this time to hold onto the integrity of your personal space ensures that you reap all the fullness this charged moment can bring. In this moment, be with yourself entirely.

1 *Drop your hands slowly to your sides. As you do so, reverse the relative positions of your hands so that the left hand, which is inside as Crossing Hands finishes, passes over the outside of the right hand.*

2 *As you move your hands, straighten your legs and stand naturally.*

3 *Carefully draw in your right heel and then your left, ending the form in the position in which you began it.*

5

TAI CHI –
THE BROADER
PICTURE

BRANCHING OUT

Tai chi is a rich art with wide applications. Many people practice all their lives for their health, while some take up the complementary art of qigung. Both systems work to maximize energy, reduce stress, and maintain health, but whereas qigung concentrates on solo practice, working with a partner is central to tai chi. Partnerwork is a way of applying the solo form of tai chi to everyday life. It creates many different situations between two people based on a rhythm of pushing and yielding, from which it becomes possible to perceive how one relates to other people. The principles of partner practice have wider applications, for they are what make tai chi a martial art.

A Chinese qigung master takes part in a psycho-physiological experiment to measure the external emission of qi or life energy from his body.

The short form has long been part of the daily routine for many people concerned with strengthening the body and the immune system. Performed regularly, it keeps the joints mobile, improves blood circulation, and stimulates breathing, and, in addition, can improve concentration, reduce anxiety and depression, and dispel insomnia. The cultivation of health is the central principle of qigung (also written "chigung" and "chi kung," see page 187), an art that is very close to tai chi but which focuses almost exclusively on stimulating the flow of chi, or life energy, around the body through exercise and control of the breath. Qigung develops strength, vitality, and stamina and can be effective in relieving chronic illness, improving debilitating disorders, and healing injuries.

Tai chi differs from qigung in a number of ways, foremost of which is the practice of exercising with a partner. Partnerwork (see pages 148–51) supports and strengthens tai chi practice by encouraging people to think about how they give, listen, and receive. This process enables them to pinpoint personal difficulties which prevent them from interacting effectively with other people. In searching for ways of overcoming problems in a class, people find a transformation taking place in their reactions to and relationships with other people.

The richness of the art of tai chi can never be experienced without exploring partnerwork. It plays

Tai chi partner practice offers great potential for self-development and transformation, as this sequence shows.

1, 2 & 3 Holding your space teaches confidence and trust. A collapsed body shape is easily upset.

1

2

3

an important role in helping people to affirm and put into perspective the qualities they are developing in their solo practice. It also helps to nurture ways of thought and action that are useful and relevant in day-to-day meetings with others. A great deal of life energy is required in everyday situations and tai chi partnerwork is designed to train people to use it wisely. While negotiating with people at work, dealing with an official, chatting with a friend, or having an argument with someone, it is important to be able to listen, respond, and hold one's space.

This process is exactly what happens in tai chi pair practice. Exchanges take place between partners in which each receives a push and gives a push in return. This is known as Pushing Hands (see pages 148–51). During this process of physical contact, patterns and habits of behavior reveal themselves. Some people, for example, tense up because they feel threatened by a push from a partner. By learning to relax physically instead of a tightening up, and also by learning to listen to another person through the medium of touch, they are able to deal with the situation without stress and to respond more freely. This carries through into their daily relationships with other people.

On the other hand, some people dislike having to push a partner in a tai chi exercise, perhaps because they were always taught that pushing is wrong. Learning to see a push as an opportunity for the partner to respond is a way of overcoming this inhibition. Some tai chi students find this a liberating experience and feel happier speaking their mind in situations where they have always felt disregarded. This is just one way in which tai chi partner practice can have a transforming effect.

The following pages explore the many branches of tai chi. People who take up tai chi for health reasons are sometimes surprised to learn that every movement, every posture in the form has an application as an evasive or attacking movement in a martial situation. There are defensive withdrawals and evasive rollbacks which, in a fight, can be used to evade a blow and regain control before moving into

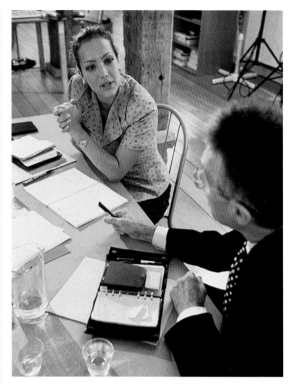

It is not surprising that listening is the first process in the cycle of tai chi partner practice - no real conversation can take place without it.

an attacking kick or punch. Partnerwork is an important part of practice for anyone who takes up tai chi as a fighting art, and pages 152–53 show pair forms relevant to its martial application.

Beginners can be surprised to find not only that tai chi is an ancient "empty hand" art, but that it extends to a number of ancient weapons arts. Pages 154–55 illustrate forms devised to develop expertise in the use of the staff and the three traditional tai chi weapons: the spear, the long sword, and the broad sword. The chapter ends with the peaceful, inward-directed qigung (pages 156–57), but even this once had a martial application in the associated neigung, an approach to the art aimed at building physical and mental resistance to blows when fighting out on a battlefield.

4, 5 & 6 Tai chi develops the ability to respond while holding your space.

WORKING WITH A PARTNER

In tai chi partnerwork two people interact in a cycle of pushing and yielding. Pushing hands offers a way of testing the solidity of movements learned in the solo form and it is a useful training technique for martial practice. Tai chi partner exercises also provide a safe, playful environment for experimenting with ways of dealing with other people. They offer possibilities for changing ingrained patterns of behavior and transforming the way one deals with people in everyday life.

Quite early on in a tai chi course many teachers introduce their students to partnerwork This consists, simply enough, of taking turns at pushing a partner and reacting to the partner's responses, and then being the one to receive and respond to the pushes. The apparent simplicity can be deceptive, however, because in partner practice, all the body structures and shapes learned in solo practice are applied.

Partnerwork follows a set of guiding principles, just as solo practice does. At the heart of these is natural way (see page 29). In partnerwork, natural way may be brought to life by

A reed in the wind is an inspiring embodiment of the qualities of tai chi natural way. With its roots embedded in the soil, it holds its space while responding to the varying pressures of the wind.

learning to respond to the partner's movements rather than finding ways of, say, dominating a situation. This is using force against force and it has no permanent benefits. Tai chi teaches the wisdom of learning to respond to the needs of the moment.

However, while recognizing the importance of responding, tai chi also teaches the principle of remaining centered and grounded. This is holding one's space. Tai chi supports this process physically and emotionally through the structure and

alignment of the body during a stance or movement.

Tai chi is not a form of psychotherapy, but it teaches the art of dealing with emotions on a physical level. For example, partner practice encourages people to look honestly at themselves. The shape or position of the body and its effectiveness in dealing with a difficult situation, such as an incoming push, is a good indicator of a person's stance in life. In exchanges of pushing and yielding, receiving and giving, there are moments when patterns of over- or under-assertiveness become clear. Tai chi guides people toward achieving a balance. Partnerwork also encourages the quality of acceptance. It is easy to suppress feelings and even experiences, and progress in tai chi depends on being able to pinpoint apprehension or anger, which manifest themselves visibly as extreme muscular tension. Recognizing and accepting such feelings is giving them the space to change. Then the energy of fear can be transformed into courage and the energy of anger might be borrowed to bring clarification.

THE POWER OF SURRENDER

A push has a life cycle. It is born, lives, runs out of momentum, and dies. Receiving is based on knowing the push will finish and not wasting energy trying to stop or deny it. Listening to and receiving the push is a way of surrendering to the situation, but it is not like waving a white flag. If your mental intention is weak when you receive the push, your body shape will be weak and caved in. A collapsed body shape is easily upset, and it makes you feel weak and vulnerable. Changing the shape

If you fall into a fast-flowing river, why waste energy struggling against the current? Surrender to its greater force, and you conserve energy you can use when an opportunity arises to reach the bank.

of your body will give you confidence and trust in yourself, and the posture will flow naturally. Think of receiving as an act of empowerment based on the natural way things work. Consciously surrendering to a situation puts you in a position of choice. To recognize and employ choice is to be empowered.

THE PROCESSES

In any tai chi partner exchange a clear sequence of events takes place as a recurring cycle, always in the same order: listening; receiving; choosing; giving. Think about how you use each of these qualities in your life.

Is each one familiar or unfamiliar, comfortable or uncomfortable? Can you find ways of incorporating a quality that feels uncomfortable into your life? If you find it difficult to receive a compliment, for instance, see if you can capture the uncomfortable moment, accept it, and replace the pattern with a different one.

1 LISTENING

This quality is at the hub of partner interaction and is carefully developed in tai chi. As if taking part in a conversation, you learn to listen through touch to the qualities (such as strength and direction) of your partner's push. As well as physical contact, the practice demands heightened sensitivity and awareness, so that you tune into your partner's intention.

2 RECEIVING

This is a deep-seated yin or feminine quality (which men need to develop as much as women). Being able to receive incoming energy enables you to neutralize it. The depth of this quality needs to match the incoming energy's force, direction, and power.

3 CHOOSING

By holding the space and surrendering to the force of the incoming push, the receiving partner has neutralized the threat and reaches a position of choice. From here the receiver can disengage; the partners can stay in contact but do nothing; or they can complete a cycle and the receiving partner clearly gives or directs the finished push back toward the other person.

4 GIVING/DIRECTING

This is a yang or masculine quality (which women need to develop as well as men). It is an energy that moves out, away from you in a clear direction, to wherever you choose to send it. It complements and balances the force of the incoming energy.

The process of listening and receiving, choosing and giving, described on the preceding two pages, are applied by employing four simple techniques. The first is touch. Through touch, an enormous amount of information can be transmitted instantly from one person to another, so touch is the technique used in tai chi to make listening possible. In tai chi touch is the basic medium for contact and communication between two people.

Sticking, the second technique, narrows the scope of touch by focusing it on a small area. One partner leads and the other tries to follow, literally without losing touch. Yang Cheng-fu, founder of the Yang tai

A flock of birds flies in formation, following a lead bird. When they turn, the whole formation turns at the same time, although there is no clear signal. When this happens it is similar to joining.

chi longform was famous for his ability to stick. It is said that a sparrow could not leave his open hand because by sticking, he could neutralize the jump the bird had to make with its legs to be able to take off. With sticking, the area of contact between two people becomes a channel for information to pass through. The point(s) of contact can move in space, but they cannot slide across each other.

Joining, by contrast, makes a leap to include the apparently non-physical. In tai chi joining happens when partners allow their feeling to extend into and envelop each other. As water fills a sponge, so joining happens with a pouring of feeling, an extending of consciousness, from one person to another.

Following is the fourth technique, and it has a unifying role. When in touch, sticking, and joined with a partner, joining prevents unnecessary action. Responding to another person instead of dictating the dialogue ensures that only essential moves are made. If one partner moves back, the follower moves forward; if the partner moves forward, the follower moves back. If the partner rests, the follower rests, listening for clues, ready to follow the next move.

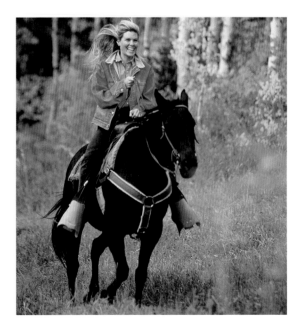

Activities like horse riding rely on communication through touch. Tai Chi develops the skill of listening and communicating by constant physical contact.

PUSHING HANDS

The techniques of touch, stick, join, follow, listen, receive, choose, and give combine in Pushing Hands to make total response possible in relating to another person.

STICKING

This is a two-person exercise, and you need to find a place to practice with enough space to move around. Begin by standing side by side. Carry out the exercise twice, for 1 to 2 minutes at a time, first with your eyes open, then with them closed, then change roles.

PRACTICING AT HOME

The techniques of pushing hands are practiced by all tai chi students, including beginners, but they cannot be learned successfully at home. Beginners learning tai chi using this book might first practice the Short Form, then with a partner seek out a teacher or attend a short introductory course that focuses on Pushing Hands. Practicing at home with a partner can then be fruitful.

PARTNER A
Rest your right palm lightly on your partner's left wrist, and when the wrist begins to move, follow it, trying to maintain the same light pressure with your palm. Wherever the wrist leads, your palm must follow.

PARTNER B
From the moment the palm of your partner's hand touches your wrist, begin to move your forearm freely but at a steady pace, and keep moving it throughout. Do not stop moving or try to escape your partner's palm.

YIELDING

This exercise can be performed solo or with one or even two partners. If there are three people, two of them push, one from either side. Practice pushing and yielding for five minutes, then change around so that everyone has a turn at pushing and at yielding.

PARTNER A
Stand comfortably with your feet a little more than one shoulder width apart, with your spine dropped slightly, and your legs bent at the knees. When your partner begins to push with one hand, yield to it by letting your spine rotate, but keep your feet firmly planted on the ground. When your partner pushes with the other hand, let your body turn the other way. Continue to yield to each push. Do not let yourself resist.

PARTNER B
Rest one hand on the shoulder and another on the back of your partner, and push steadily with one hand. Now push with the other hand, and continue in this way, pushing alternately with one hand, then with the other.

A FIGHTING ART

For much of its long history tai chi has been a respected fighting art. Its martial forms are thought to have evolved centuries ago from "external" or "hard" arts – rather like today's karate or kung fu – into an "internal" art, founded on inner strength and concentration. The change is said to have been made by the legendary Taoist sage Chang San-feng, who, it is related, saw a fight between a snake and a bird. Struck by the ability of snake and bird to yield, so that neither could overcome the other, Chang modified his hard fighting art to a "softer" one, in which attack might come from withdrawal, and defense might be based on neutralizing blows instead of using hard force.

Every tai chi posture has a martial application, so the body makes the same graceful shapes in the martial applications of the art.

To apply the principles of tai chi to fighting takes study and a great deal of dedication, and many people who begin tai chi do not expect to learn to fight. There are teachers in the West who try to deny that tai chi is a martial art at all, claiming it to be a set of exercises to maintain health with no fighting application. Yet the historic role of tai chi on the battlefield and in civil insurrections (see pages 20–23) has been well documented.

Learning a form is always the first stage of tai chi, so people may not begin learning a martial application until they have spent some months practicing a solo form (see pages 84–143) and have progressed to partnerwork (see pages 148–51, and opposite). People are often motivated to branch out by a desire to add a dimension to tai chi practice more than by an interest in learning to fight. In fact, everyone could benefit from seeing how each posture can be adapted to a martial situation. It clarifies the intention behind the postures and it brings focus to their practice. It is obvious how a punch or a kick might be applied in a fight, but the martial role of a posture such as Diagonal Flying or Golden Rooster Stands on One Leg may not be so clear. A good teacher will always be able to demonstrate the martial forms of the postures.

In fact, tai chi strikes a perfect balance between the expression of yang or masculine aggression and the development of the yin quality of inner softness. All tai chi students – women and men – need to learn to express yang energy. Little can be achieved, internally in practice or externally against an opponent, with a wavering, unfocused kick. Tai chi is sometimes misinterpreted as an evasive martial art based on defence and not attack. It is, however, as aggressive as it needs to be. There is no mistaking the impact of a forceful punch.

And men who study tai chi, as well as women, need to understand how to neutralize or absorb an incoming force, when and how to give way in order to conserve energy, and how the hidden face of yielding is attack. The martial intent behind the posture Withdraw and Push, for example, then becomes clear. Cultivating the true martial spirit is as much about self-development as it is about self-defence.

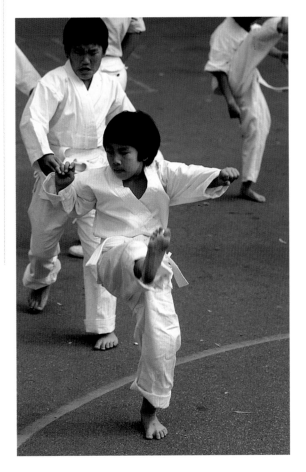

The practice of yield and attack postures greatly benefits tai chi as a fighting art.

A PAIR FORM

The principles of partner practice are the basis of tai chi as a fighting art, so understanding Pushing Hands is central to the sequences illustrated here, which are typical of the stages through which you might be taught the martial form of Tai Chi. It involves learning to apply each of the eight basic postures (Ward off, Rollback, Press, Push, Pull, Split, Elbow, and Shoulder - see pages 66–7) in a variety of situations. People are sometimes surprised to discover that unless you go on to free fighting (see below), learning tai chi as a fighting art may never involve combat with a partner.

Partner exercises train you to be fully present. They dissolve anticipation, teaching you to focus on what is happening and deal with it, rather than imagine what might happen. Pushing Hands in martial arts practice involves learning many different partner exercises. Some are choreographed, some improvised, and there are others with fixed and moving steps. Through them you learn perfect theoretical responses to imagined situations. Once you have learned the basic moves in Single and Double Pushing Hands, illustrated below, you can improvise instead of following a set pattern. Free Pushing trains you to understand when different techniques are most appropriate.

SINGLE PUSHING HANDS

This exercise develops basic listening, sticking, and yielding skills, and is often used as an introduction to partner exercises. You and your partner stand facing each other in a bow and arrow stance with the palm and wrist of your left or right hand in contact. You alternately push and receive in a continuous cycle.

DOUBLE PUSHING HANDS

This extension of Single Pushing Hands, using both hands instead of just one, offers more possibilities. The illustration shows part of the Wardoff, Rollback, Press, and Push sequence of Pushing Hands.

FREE PUSHING

Students familiar with the basic principles of yielding and neutralizing in partnerwork are then given the opportunity to try free pushing – you do not know whether your partner will push or yield. Free pushing makes it possible to apply any of the eight basic postures and respond in a more spontaneous way.

DA LU ("BIG ROLLBACK")

This choreographed movement is first learned as a solo form, then put together with a partner. It develops the ability to step and move while applying hand techniques. There are many forms of Da Lu, the one shown here is common in Cheng Man-ch'ing style.

SAN SHOU

The San Shou is what is known as a fast form. It is an advanced form, usually taught only to students after 3 years' practice. It is learned as two solo forms which are the two sides to a choreographed piece for two players. As a solo practice, the speed at which it runs highlights the many circles, spirals, and centrifugal forces not so easily felt in the ordinary form. With a partner it develops agility and response ability.

FREE FIGHTING

A few people who are especially interested and wish to take part in martial arts competitions go on to free fighting. It is an advanced form, and students must know the solo form. They may spend time learning a longer form and advanced techniques of partner practice and free pushing. As a safety precaution, some people pad up with protective gear and really test their fighting skills.

TAI CHI WEAPONS FORMS

Some people shy away from learning a weapon form, perceiving it as aggressive. However, although the tai chi sword and spear once saw violent service on the battlefield, in tai chi practice today they are employed as a means of improving agility and alertness, and never in combat with a partner. Beneath the initial reaction, however, may lie a deeper truth: that seeing or handling a weapon puts people in touch with an inner discomfort about their aggression. The fearless warrior spirit hungers for this discomfort, and, seeking to meet it head-on, plunges into the frightening arena of weapons arts.

Warrior or not, learning to use the tai chi battlefield weapons develops skills and qualities in everyone, woman or man, which are as relevant at the corporation negotiating table as they are to running a household. A bonus of moving into this branch of tai chi is that as well as learning to wield a weapon, students study a solo form. Learning its principles takes about a year, and after that, choreographed parries and thrusts may also be practiced in partnerwork. The martial exercises have the effect of deepening understanding of the postures and movements in the solo form, and for this reason alone many people decide to extend their experience of tai chi by trying a weapon form.

Although each weapon form develops a slightly different set of skills and qualities, all highlight aspects of the open hand form. Broadly speaking they also all heighten coordination, focus, balance, and mental alertness.

Weapons practice also raises the body's energy levels and channels the energy outward. This higher throughput of energy cleanses and clears the body, as if it were burning off rubbish. It balances the temperament. It invites people who tend to be inward-directed to extend outward, and those who are normally outgoing learn how to anchor themselves inwardly.

The weapons arts all put more emphasis on mastering of the outflow of energy than do the open hands forms. Intention, mind, and energy (chi) all need to reach the tip of the weapon and extend beyond it.

Partnerwork with weapons develops alertness of spirit and deft footwork.

This solo posture of Tai Chi, using a long sword, is called Drifting With The Current.

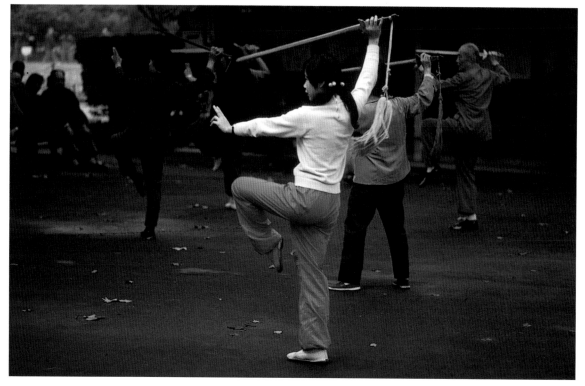

A tai chi student in Shanghai practices with the jian or long sword, balancing carefully and directing the attention outward.

THE LONG SWORD

The tai chi sword, called the long sword, straight sword or jian, is the weapon most commonly associated with the practice of tai chi. In China it is known as the weapon of the scholar and the gentleman, because its use embraces the same basic principles as Chinese calligraphy. Sword and brush are controlled in a similar way, with the attention focused on the tip. The tai chi sword is said to have been used as a tool by Taoist sages and is described in Chinese mythology as having magical powers. It is a weapon of great sensitivity and is generally considered the most subtle and the hardest to learn, requiring swiftness, deft footwork, flexibility, and sharpness of spirit.

THE BROAD SWORD

It is said that the broad sword or dao can be learned in 100 days, whereas the straight sword takes 10,000. There lies the difference. The broad sword is a slashing weapon that uses large, circular, sweeping movements, generating considerable force from a relaxed center. Two types of broad sword are clearly distinguishable. One is a heavyweight version that could double as an agricultural machete and was once the choice of farming people. The other is a lightweight, military version which is sharper and swifter. It is a good weapon for practice as it mobilizes the spine and torso.

THE SPEAR

The characteristic movements of the spear are strong, linear, well-extended thrusts joined with deflections. Repeated practice is said to develop fa jing – the ability to release energy to send an opponent flying. The clear, masculine or yang movements develop clarity and decisiveness.

THE STAFF

The staff is more commonly associated with the hard or external fighting forms developed at the Shaolin Temple and monastery in southern China, the birthplace of Chinese martial arts as long ago as the 600s. However, the tai chi schools also developed staff forms, as the principles of the art can be put into practice with a staff just as with a sword or spear. Some staff forms evolved directly from the spear. It is said that in the 19th century Yang Ban-hou, son of the founder of the Yang style, ordered the heads to be removed from all spears after his daughter was killed during a spear practice session.

CAMOUFLAGED WEAPONS

In the past it was not always possible to carry a weapon in China. At certain times and in certain places weapons have been banned. But objects of daily use, such as canes used as walking sticks, and fans, could double as practical aids to self-defense. Training in one of these forms grew out of a need for a weapon that allowed people to go about their daily business confident that they were equipped to meet an assault.

CULTIVATING ENERGY

Qigung (or chi kung) is an approach to exercise that complements tai chi. In fact the two are so closely related that some teachers practice what they call "tai chi qigung." Posture, movement, breathing, visualization, meditation, and focus are central to both, and both are health-giving exercises. But whereas tai chi emphasizes partner practice and has martial applications, qigung is largely a solo practice with less emphasis on interaction with others. Qigung means "energy work" and, essentially, it focuses on cultivating chi or life energy to promote well-being and vitality. Like tai chi, however, qigung encourages self-development.

Like tai chi, qigung is good to practice in a clear, clean and bright environment, either in or out of doors.

Because tai chi and qigung are so similar, they are often confused. (Qigung is the modern spelling; the term has traditionally been written in many different ways, most commonly "chigung" or "chi kung," see page 184.) This art is commonly defined as exercises for health, and tai chi is sometimes explained as movements for fighting. Both definitions betray a limited perception of the two arts. Tai chi is also a healing art (see pages 24–5) and qigung can teach how

to conserve and focus energy in martial training. By contrast with the flow of movement of tai chi, qigung tends to be more static. Internally, however, it seeks to build and move energy. It is said to be "inward-building," that is, it charges the body's energy source and tones it up physically. Tai chi, by contrast, draws energy from the body and directs it outward through pushing hands and weapons forms.

Qigung and tai chi have evolved from common origins now buried deep in antiquity. Through the ages qigung has evolved into many different styles and approaches. For example, neigung is called the art of internal power because its emphasis is on developing the body's internal energy through exercises, postures, breathing, and visualization. It was once called upon to harden the body for battle by training it to tolerate blows. Adepts described how training would begin by gently striking the body's vital points with a small bag of Chinese beans, and progress to blows of increasing force with larger and heavier implements. Today, neigung is used to strengthen confidence in pushing hands or fighting practice, and to deepen relaxation.

Tai chi and qigung complement each other perfectly and are often taught together. Qigung exercises are often used to prepare for the tai chi form (see pages 76–81). Tai chi qigung exploits the similarities between the two to develop energy-building techniques. For example, a tai chi posture might be held for five minutes to build energy, or treated as a solo exercise and repeated many times to work the muscles and speed the circulation of the blood.

Qigung is primarily concerned with health and it has developed many exercises aimed at directing the mind and the life force to the organs, the joints, and other parts of the body to promote health. This is its value, for its own sake and as a solo practice to support tai chi.

Many types of qigung are practiced today. Indeed, the way the tai chi form has been presented in this book, with the use of visualization, could be said to take a qigung approach. Opposite is a short qigung sequence that can be practiced on its own or can be added to the preparation exercises on pages 76–81.

CENTERING

Begin each exercise standing with your weight distributed evenly and your feet one shoulder width apart. Spend a few minutes softening and opening each reference point (see page 63).

EARTH BREATHING

This exercise relaxes and the working of the legs and arms stimulates circulation. Imagine yourself breathing the earth inward, filling your body from toes to crown. Tune into the rhythm of your breath, imagining it activating and clearing the energy centers. The out-breath releases unwanted energy and returns you to the earth.

1 *Bring all your weight onto your right leg, and sit deeply into it. Slide your left foot forward, lifting the heel slightly.*

2 *Feel connected to the earth. Breathe in deeply, and as you do so, slowly rise by straightening your right leg, and let your arms float up.*

3 *Breathe out naturally while sitting your weight deeply into your right leg and lowering your hands to the lower tantien.*

4 *Repeat steps 1–3 at least two more times before transferring your weight to the left leg and repeating them three times on the left side.*

5 *Transfer your weight back to the right leg and repeat the cycle on the right side, bringing your arms out to the sides and raising and lowering them in step 2 in the manner of slow-motion flying. Repeat the cycle once more on the left leg. Finish by centering.*

SUNRISE

This exercise lightens and refreshes the spirit.

1 *Sit deeply into both feet and very slowly raise your hands to chest level, imagining that you lift the sun from under the earth up through your feet.*

2 *Imagine the sun fills your heart and that its light fills your whole body and bursts out to shine in the space around you. Raise your hands and your face toward the sky.*

3 *Relax your face and turn forward, and, lowering your arms, open them fully so they extend upward and outward. Enjoy this position of radiance.*

4 *Finish by centering, then repeat steps 1–3 twice.*

SUNSET

This position leaves you feeling quiet, contained, and peaceful. Its gathering and calming moves complement the upward and outward energy of Sunrise, above.

1 *Circle your arms upward in a large arc, finishing with your fingertips about 2 inches apart opposite your face. Respond with a sense of gathering.*

2 *Move your hands slowly and gracefully down to rest by your sides like the sun setting.*

3 *Repeat steps 1 and 2 two more times, then rest your hands on the lower tantien. Imagine all your energy centers alive and balanced.*

6

TAI CHI
FOR CREATIVE
LIVING

TAI CHI FOR LIFE

To move with grace, power, and beauty, to harmonize with the heartbeat, the breath, and the cosmos is to receive the greatest gifts tai chi can offer. Yet practicing the movements can take as little as ten minutes, and although that can be stretched to a two-hour session, what about the rest of the day? Tai chi is not an art that need be restricted to "training," or imprisoned in a time slot. It should never become a treadmill activity that dulls the imagination. It is a creative activity which, allowed to extend beyond practice into everyday life, will invigorate the mind and enrich the spirit.

It is important to be aware of the body's evolving daily needs, but not always easy at first to know what they are. Try clearing the mind of daily preoccupations and respond spontaneously. You might suddenly feel like turning the spine or expressing all your energy in a kick.

Beginners often ask how much they need to practice. The short answer is that at the beginning it is a good idea to aim at practicing for about 10 minutes a day. Without practice it is difficult to improve, and for steady improvement it is important to practice regularly. However, it is equally necessary to have the right approach to discipline. To force oneself to practice is to adopt a rigid, over-zealous approach, and although commitment is essential, so is inspiration. A child will play day after day with enviable self-discipline and marked absorption. But if a child were made to play for so long at a certain time every day, the commitment would be enforced and the absorption would, no doubt, dissipate. The point is that practice must be based on intuition, feeling, and common sense, for to be fruitful tai chi needs to be practiced with passion.

The movements of tai chi embody the Taoist principles on which it is based, and the idea behind practice is to bring these

Spontaneity is as essential to tai chi practice as it is to a child's play.

to life. They are simple: tai chi expresses the polarity of opposites – yin and yang, open and closed, full and empty, and central balance (see pages 26–7) – and the dynamic equilibrium between them.

One way of keeping practice alive is to make one pair of polarities or one quality the theme of the day or the week, observing it at work when practicing the simplest movements, and noticing how one quality, such as listening, feels in relation to its opposite. It is easy to extend the idea of exploring a quality beyond practice by observing different aspects of it as they occur in daily life, noticing one's own habits of listening or failing to listen during interactions with other people, and observing how and when they listen. Eventually it becomes second nature to explore the qualities in daily life, noticing links between their appearance in different situations and in tai chi movements. Which movements seem to enhance listening? Do they feel familiar and comfortable, or difficult? Exercises of this kind can be more effective than trying to make the quality work in practice. Their effect can be to sharpen the awareness.

Nevertheless, learning the form does mean attending regular, disciplined practice sessions for as long as a year, and it is important during this time not to lose sight of personal needs. This is where free practice and freestyle movement (see pages 164–5) are

Practicing tai chi overlooked by the Temple of Heaven in Beijing.
Daily practice works, not because it is the correct thing to do but
because mind and body together respond to it.

most valuable. The mind and body are constantly changing. One day there may be a need for grounding, and another may bring a need to move faster, or to direct the attention outward. People evolve ways of finding out what type of practice suits them best.

To acknowledge tai chi as a practice that affects the health of body, mind, and soul is to open to the broad range of experiences it offers. Exercising is only one aspect of practice; there is more to tai chi than that. Some of its many avenues are explored in the following pages. The experiences provided by each one furnish inspiration for practice, keeping its spirit alive and giving creativity a channel for expression.

KITCHEN PRACTICE

One excellent way of extending practice time is always to have a couple of possibilities up your sleeve. Perhaps you want to develop a stepping technique or get a better sense of how your spine turns. Then, those endless minutes when coffee is warming or bread toasting stand out as ideal times for practice (just watch out for burned toast). In a slow line at a checkout, practice feeling weight transfer from one foot to the other. In your car in a traffic gridlock, breathe more deeply, become centered, massage your hands. There are countless possibilities for practice. Any time you find yourself waiting, think of it as another opportunity.

NATURE AND THE ELEMENTS

In traditional Chinese philosophy the five elements – water, wood, fire, metal, and earth – are thought of as the basis of all life on earth, and for hundreds of years Western philosophy saw the universe as composed of earth, water, fire, and air. Even without the guidance of philosophy it is easy to see how these elements are the raw materials of nature. Tai chi is a system of movement that follows the natural way of things, so practicing tai chi must involve learning about nature and about ourselves, for the self is a fundamental part of nature. The study of tai chi is an investigation into the very essence of life.

The concept of the elements is central to all Chinese healing arts, including acupuncture and moxibustion, and Chinese herbal medicine.

Everyone seems to have an unconscious familiarity and sense of ease with one or perhaps two of the elements. Many people, for example, would agree that a solid, thickset, steady person could be said to be earthy, and a lightly built person is more like air or fire. The language is full of expressions that derive from the ancient concept of the elements. People with a vivid imagination are often described as air-headed, and we talk of fiery tempers. Each of the four elements has its distinctive characteristics.

The objective of working with the elements is to widen the understanding of their qualities beyond what is familiar, to recognize your own elemental qualities, and to encourage people to experience working with the elements in many different ways. A naturally earthy person can experience how it feels to

be light, and a light person can discover the solid nature of earth as a real physical experience. This exploration of elemental qualities can be exciting. It is like adding more pieces to the jigsaw of personal life. It extends the breadth and quality of individual experience and adds new possibilities to the range of responses you can bring to daily encounters with nature and other people.

The exercises shown here present a contrast between discoveries you can make in the immediate environment, and inspiration to be drawn from nature. The fruits of every investigation into the elements can then be brought back into the tai chi form. Discovering how it feels to move in a light, airy way, a solid, earthy way, a flowing, watery way, or an energetic, fiery way enhances practice and makes it more enjoyable.

DISCOVERING THE ELEMENTS

The elements are everywhere, and in these exercises you learn to recognize them and to embody their qualities in movement. This is a creative and rewarding process because it uses the power of the imagination to create tangible effects. The qualities of the elements can be embodied through the tai chi postures or in free movement (see pages 164–5). The following exercise shows you how to do this through visualization.

VISUALIZATION

The aim of the visualizations is to enable you to implement the energy of the different elements. During visualization you should sit, stand, or lie down, as you feel appropriate. Search your imagination for an image related to the subject, giving it time to find the image that exactly expresses your feelings or needs of the moment. When visualizing fire, for instance, you might

imagine a cosy log fire, or a furnace. Once you have found an appropriate image, examine it closely until you can almost feel it. Imagine its essence penetrating the cells of your body so you become part of it. Spend all the time you need to incorporate the image into your body. Afterward, notice what difference it has made as you move in tai chi or go about your daily business.

ELEMENT: EARTH

Associated qualities: Rootedness, steadiness, groundedness, solidity, strength, stability.
Visualization: Call to mind anything earthy – a mountain, freshly tilled soil, an animal such as an elephant or a Shire horse.

ELEMENT: FIRE

Associated qualities: Energy, warmth, light, joy, comfort, speed, cleansing, transformation, decisiveness.
Visualization: This may be sunshine, the glowing embers of a camp fire, or lightning.

ELEMENT: WATER

Associated qualities: Relaxation, power, knowing your place, ease, effortlessness, no wasting of energy, tirelessness, flow, movement, fearlessness, simplicity, change.
Visualization: This may be anything from a lake to a raindrop, from the calm sea to a raging torrent.

ELEMENT: AIR

Associated qualities: Lightness, sensitivity, feeling, alertness, communicability, clarity, swift change.
Visualization: Think of the different aspects of air, from soft, warm, scented night air to a harsh, cold, wintry blast.

INSPIRATION FROM NATURE

Pictures and records show that all through human history people have sought to fulfil a need for communication with nature. The Taoists are remembered today more for their study of nature than for other aspects of their philosophy.

To draw inspiration from nature is to experience something of the essence of life. The following exercises explore different ways of communing with nature.

1 *Go to a wild place where the elements seem raw and clear. You may know a river you can go to sit beside, or a hillside or an outcrop of rock you can lie on. Wild places are no longer plentiful, so you may need to plan this exercise as if it were a pilgrimage of a day or longer. Go camping somewhere you can light a camp fire, take a trip to a wild area of coast.*

2 *When you arrive, swim in the river or the sea, feel the wind and rain on your skin, watch the clouds. Look and listen, absorbing the teachings of nature. Understand how nature works. Notice the interaction between all the elements in creating life.*

ELEMENTS IN URBAN LIFE

The elements are all around in cities and built areas, and in cultivated countryside. Notice how the water behaves when you are bathing or showering. Stand by an open window and feel the air with your hands, on your face, and when you breathe. Stand outdoors and face the sunshine, closing your eyes and feeling its warmth and light. At any moment of any day it is possible to awaken your life with elemental awareness.

CREATING A SPECIAL PLACE

Create a special place in your home for a collection of objects symbolic of the elements. A rock you came across one day, a feather, a bowl of water just from the faucet, and a candle can create a strongly elemental and beautiful atmosphere to keep you in contact with nature.

A word of warning: enjoy the exercise, but take great care: light fires only where they are not prohibited and will do no harm, and make certain they are protected from spreading and completely extinguished when you leave. Swim only where it is safe, and never alone. Stand in the wind only where you are not in danger.

FREESTYLE MOVEMENT

Everyone knows how to move, but few adults are aware that, as they have matured, the range of movements of which they are capable has steadily decreased. Moreover, many people's movements are restricted to a narrow band of activity – sitting on a chair, lying, standing to work at tasks, walking – and they have forgotten altogether how to move freely, as if that were something better left to athletes. Freestyle movement arrests this decline by recalling the range of movements natural to children. Performing movements that lie outside the normal boundaries of the form loosens up the body and dissolves inhibitions, bringing deeper understanding and increased vitality to the more disciplined movements of the tai chi form.

Although at first it might seem easy to move without the restrictions of form, it can be hard to know where to begin. A good starting point is to remember the Taoist principles of tai chi. Freestyle movement might equally be termed Radical Taoist Movement, because it is based on the seven basic qualities of yin and yang, open and closed, full and empty, and central equilibrium (see pages 26–7). It develops these polarities as human qualities, exploring them in movement.

The aim of freestyle movement is to restore the ease of movement which is the natural human condition. For many people, simple sequences of movement, such as progressing from sitting to standing, standing to lying, lying to crawling, which small children perform with ease and which are everyone's birthright, have become for many people a major exertion, causing great discomfort. In recent years a fashion has emerged for aerobic activities and working out on machines in gyms, indicating an awareness of the need to widen the body's regular range of movements. But that type of training tends to exercise just one particular part of the body.

Tai chi treats body and mind as a single unit, and the exercises on these pages are designed to stimulate the body to restore free, holistic movement. These introductory exercises are, however, just a set of guidelines to enable people to overcome their initial misgivings about moving and begin to enjoy movement for movement's sake. Real power develops when the beginner abandons the core exercises and begins to improvise and explore, developing themes and launching into new experiences in movement.

Freestyle movement is not intended to be an alternative to tai chi, but to support it in the sense that it provides a forum for exploring and developing the basic principles of the art in an unrestricted way. It works on the physical and mental impediments that slow progress in learning the form, so it is important to take regular notice of what free movement contributes to formal practice. It means moving according to the principles at the hub of Taoist thinking and at the core of tai chi, and its effect is to bring meaning to the postures and empower the individual to move more exactly.

1 *Move into an open shape, then into a closed shape, taking careful notice of how different the two polarities feel. Repeat these movements, but this time, as you perform an open movement try to feel a little more open; and as you move into a closed position try to close yourself a little further. Notice the polarity increasing and the dynamic energy growing. Repeat the moves several times, always trying to take each polarity a little further.*

2 *Now add a second set of polarities, large and small, say. Try to define what happens. Explore different combinations: large and open; large and closed; small and open; small and closed. Then add another polarity. Continue this exploration until you feel like finishing, then continue with new polarities in another session.*

RADICAL TAOIST MOVEMENT

Before you begin to move, pause and focus on one of the polarities. Open and closed is used as an example here, but you could choose light and heavy, fast and slow; awareness directed outward, awareness directed inward; or any other pair of polarities. Follow the guidelines below, and you will soon begin to move in a way that is alive, real, and fun. This is exploring radical Taoist movement, journeying through a landscape of experiences, some of which feel familiar and comfortable, others strange and rather disturbing. Expect occasionally to feel surprisingly comfortable with an unfamiliar movement.

EASE OF MOVEMENT

Your body moves on three levels: the horizontal – lying or perhaps rolling; the semi-upright – crawling, sitting, perhaps crouching or squatting; and the vertical – standing, walking, running, and so on. These movements reflect the evolution of human mobility from infant to adult, and the exercises take you progressively from the first to the last, exploring the potential for movement of each stage. Work on a pattern of moving and resting, and occasionally stretching out. Breathe deeply and do not hold your breath when moving. Let your breathing complement your body shapes and movements.

When you feel at ease with these movements, try exploring and developing themes. Run through the basic sequence and then improvise, letting the practice unfold.

CRAWLING AND SITTING

Lie on your back and lift your head and then your shoulders and trunk until you are in a sitting position. You will notice that you need to exert a great deal of muscular effort and tension to do this. Now lie on your back again, and this time roll over to the left while drawing in your right knee and you will find yourself in a crawling position almost without effort. Spend some time crawling, then experiment with lowering your hips until you find a sitting position. Practice this exercise a number of times, easing your way as effortlessly as you can between lying and crawling and sitting. While you do so, notice what use you make of your arms and hips. Think about how it feels to roll and crawl and sit. Does it bring any memories into mind?

LYING AND ROLLING

STANDING AND WALKING

Whenever you move between the three basic levels, think of moving with ease and fluidity, not in straight lines but in circles and spirals. When you are ready, spiral your way from sitting into a standing position, then back to a sitting position. Repeat this movement many times until you feel comfortable with it. Then, perhaps on a different occasion, experiment with walking and other types of vertical movement: skipping, hopping, jumping, running, and combinations of these. Always look for ease in movement.

Lie in a clean, comfortable place where you can let yourself relax completely. Spend as much time as you feel you want to in this wonderful, restorative position. When you are ready, roll over and, if you feel you want to, roll over the ground. Rest after moving if you feel you need to. While lying and while rolling, think about how it feels to have your body close to the earth.

CREATIVITY AND EXPRESSION

Creativity is the expression of inspirations, thoughts and ideas in ways that range from exploring relationships with other people to dance and sports, and making or doing things with the hands. People often say they are not creative, but this is more an expression of lack of confidence than of the truth. The primal force of creation is sexual energy, and that is what brought us here. To live fully is to express this primal energy in the same way that the universe creates cycles of birth, life, and death. There is also a strong link between creativity, expression, and life energy. To cultivate this aspect of tai chi is to create a channel through which one's buried creative urges can surface.

Creativity springs from the urge to express. It begins with the natural outward expression of inner feelings, and from there often springs a desire to communicate emotion in singing or playing music, or in poetry, perhaps. Children are naturally uninhibited, but as they mature, they learn to suppress certain feelings. It is now well understood that in the more northern cultures generally, emotions tend to be more repressed than in southern areas, and that in certain north European societies especially, men find it difficult to address their feelings.

To inhibit one's natural expression creates stress, and in extreme cases stress replaces expression. When the body is stressed, tension builds in the muscles in response to a perceived danger. This stress mechanism is now very well known: the body prepares for fight or flight by gathering energy. Hormones, such as adrenaline, are released which increase the blood pressure, speed up the heart, and increase the breathing rate. When the situation calls for physical action, such as fleeing, this energy is utilized, and the hormone production subsides, but when the danger takes the form of a frightening bank statement or a crisis in a relationship, the gathered energy remains unused and the hormones continue to circulate. If stressful situations recur day after day, year after year, hormones build up in the bloodstream, stress becomes chronic, and these factors may cause uncomfortable symptoms, leading to illnesses as serious as stroke, heart disease, and perhaps even cancer.

One simple way of preventing the development of chronic stress is to eliminate its causes; another is to change one's reaction to those

Dance is a powerful medium for the physical expression of creativity.

causes. People often find that talking about their problems can be instrumental in clearing the mental and emotional reasons for the stress. The cycle of tension and adrenaline build-up in the body can be broken through treatment such as massage and exercise.

Tai chi is a holistic practice which works at all levels to prevent the build-up of tension, break the stress cycle, relieve symptoms, and so prevent illness from developing. It generates energy in the hui yin and lower tantien energy centers (see pages 54–7), which rises as part of a cycle that moves to the top of the head and down to the pelvis. This energy tries to find an outlet, and people often feel stifled in the throat and chest if they deny the powerful and natural urge to express it, perhaps through an outlet for creativity. Tai chi also has a massaging effect on mind and body, so it works against the build-up of chronic tension. After practice, the root cause of tension can often be seen, heard, remembered, and felt. Once it has become apparent, it can be dealt with.

Acting is a way of expressing emotion and communicating it to other actors and to the wider audience.

The causes of stress are therefore more likely to become clear if occasionally after tai chi practice a space is made for self-expression. This involves sitting quietly or lying down to rest and waiting in a receptive way. Images, thoughts, memories, and feelings swirl into consciousness, and at first one may be able to do little more than acknowledge them, notice them, and give them time to make their way to the surface. Eventually, it may be possible to recognize a pattern which may be interpreted as a message from the unconscious, or to find ways of harnessing the energy being restrained by some form of personal inhibition.

Creative expression is one way of utilizing the energy generated by tai chi and people often discover a heartfelt need to continue with the drawing they abandoned years ago, or to buy a new camera, to join a choir, or audition for a part in a play. There are many different forms of expression. One person might decide to have a child; another to travel for a while. Someone else might decide to take the plunge and set up a business. In the case studies described on pages 178–83 there are several examples of a search for creativity which has surfaced through tai chi and found its eventual expression.

THE NEED FOR SELF-EXPRESSION

Before you find the right form of self-expression, you may experience uncertainty and confusion, or physical symptoms of frustration, such as a choking feeling during certain postures. At this point, bear in mind that speaking is one of the simplest, most accessible, and natural forms of self-expression. If you find it hard to express your feelings, see if you can find an outlet through your voice. Begin by listening to it – if you are telling someone about an anxiety, notice how your body feels before, during, and after your talk. If you are familiar with expressing your feelings, try experimenting with your voice in creative ways – through play and poetry readings, public speaking, imitating other voices, or singing. The effect of self-expression through the voice is not to be underestimated.

THE CREATIVITY CYCLE

Enlivened practice stirs creative energy and the need to express it.

As the flow develops, blocks to creativity dissolve.

Good health enlivens the approach to practice, so that body and mind are stimulated.

Releasing creativity raises the levels of life force energy circulating around the body.

Increased life energy becomes a strong healing force, which generates health.

Overcoming inhibitions to the expression of thoughts and feelings through tai chi releases a stream of energy to flow outward.

TAI CHI AT WORK

People these days lead very busy lives and have little time to spare for interests such as tai chi. It is worth while, however, finding a way of fitting a class and practice time into a weekly schedule, however packed it may be. Learning to be flexible is an important part of a holistic approach to health. Tai chi is an investment which will pay dividends in a calmer outlook, improved concentration, and a feeling of greater control over the events of the day. Better time management begins with making time for daily practice.

In the industrial societies of today, time pressure begins for many people at school or college. Students often have trouble fitting in course work with home study, school or college activities, relationships, and hobbies or interests. For working people the business day seems to lengthen relentlessly, with the pressure of getting ready for meetings and traveling to conferences, getting through the workload, and catching up on all the new developments. Workers double as parents, and parents have jobs as well as families. And where once working life ended at an early retirement age, many people need to work for longer, or they fill their retirement years with voluntary work. These pages offer guidelines for anyone who despairs at the prospect of finding ten minutes a day to practice tai chi.

Before making any plans it is essential to be convinced that tai chi will be worth all the effort. The decision must not spring from a sense of duty ("I ought to get more exercise;" or "I really ought to do it for my health.") but from a yearning to give something to yourself, from an inner desire to learn tai chi. Practice must be

In a life whose every moment is planned and scheduled in advance, finding time for tai chi is a way of building space into your life, giving some thought to the needs of your mind and body, loving yourself for a few minutes a day.

something every learner looks forward to. It must never be enforced, never an activity that has to be stuck to because you have made a promise to yourself. Resolving to join a class made at the New Year is hardly likely to result in steady, sustained progress. To advance in tai chi and to achieve the lasting benefits practice can give, it is necessary to dig more deeply into the self than that.

The health benefits of long-term practice are reviewed on pages 24–5. In addition, tai chi shows people ways of dealing with the tensions and stresses of working life, and how to maintain an equilibrium so that concentration, relationships both at work and outside it, do not suffer, and well-being is maintained.

Tai chi can be equally beneficial to people whose time is not always in demand. People who are unemployed, people who for a wide range of reasons find it hard to fill their day, and people, such as single parents and people working at home alone, who are busy but isolated, might all find a new satisfaction and inspiration to guide their lives from a class or from a commitment to practice tai chi at home.

A real desire to learn tai chi comes from deep inside, from self-love. This is a form of energy responsible for the wellbeing of body, mind, heart, and soul. Everyone needs to give self-love the time and space to blossom. Anyone who is truly motivated to make time for tai chi in their life can be confident that their commitment will work out because it is based on inspiration and not on enforced discipline.

Anyone caring for a family full-time can benefit especially from partnerwork and pushing hands, which explore relationships and enable you to develop new ways of dealing with people.

MAKING A CHOICE

Perhaps you have been thinking of beginning tai chi, but you are not sure you have time for it. Perhaps you have tried it out and would like to devote more time to it. Any ongoing commitment involves planning and the following five questions are designed to help you reach a decision. The most important question in the list is the second one. If the answer is no, go no farther. If the answer is yes, you can be sure that it comes from a part of you in touch with your needs, the part of you that knows how to look after yourself. It is worthwhile pausing to think about this for a few minutes.

With this knowledge as a foundation, you are now in a position to take practical steps to implement your decision. Be easy with yourself – set comfortably attainable targets for the amount of time you need to practice, so that it is valued time. Two minutes of really focused practice can be enough to ensure the success of your day.

1 Is my life so busy that I do not have time to exercise?
2 Do I want to change?
3 What do I need to change to create time for tai chi?
4 How much time do I need each day?
5 How will I implement this change?

For anyone whose daily schedule seems to have empty spaces, tai chi can provide a focus in the day, maintain health, raise vitality, and restore a sense of purpose and self-worth.

A PRACTICAL APPROACH TO EXERCISE

It can be helpful to create your own exercise program based on the time you have available and the type of exercise you want. This program is based on a 10-minute schedule (to the end of step 7) or an extended 12-minute schedule, and it is a compilation of some of the exercises in parts 3 and 4.

	EXERCISE	DURATION	WHERE TO FIND IT
2	Turning With Feet	1 minute	page 76
3	Rainbow Circle	2 minutes	page 77
4	Snake Shake your whole body from top to toe, including hands and fingers	30 seconds	page 80
5	Push as a Key Move posture in a repeating cycle of back, down, and forward	2 minutes	page 75

6	Massage your hands
	   " " face
	   " " ears
		30 seconds
		30 seconds
		30 seconds
			page 25
			"
			"

7	Beginning posture	2 minutes	pages 86–7
8	Ward Off Left, Ward Off Right, Rollback, Press, Push, and Single Whip	2 minutes	pages 88–95

TAI CHI AT LEISURE

Tai chi is the main recreation of many people, but for an increasing number it is being taken up as a valuable supplement to a major sport, such as golf or basketball. Tai chi exercises the whole body, emphasizes posture, balance, and energy management, and it develops body awareness and mental alertness, and these qualities are in high demand for greater enjoyment and success in a number of other activities. These pages show how tai chi can be the perfect backup to improving performance in sports ranging from horse-riding to soccer, but it can be equally valuable in increasing success in more sedentary interests, from poker to pool to playing the guitar.

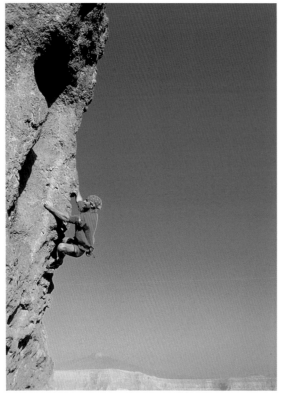

Rock-climbing defies gravity, while tai chi keeps the feet firmly planted on the ground, yet there are common links.

It is now a truism that a comfortably relaxed body works better, and it follows that relaxing will improve performance in almost any activity, physical or mental. Tai chi teaches how to dispel tension and control energy flow, and these qualities are now being used by professionals in a number of sports to improve concentration and the ability to relax during moments of great tension.

Every aspect of tai chi can be useful preparation for other physical activities. The preparatory exercises, for example (see pages 76–81), are an excellent way of warming up. Some people select five or six exercises that seem to answer their needs of the moment, whereas others will run through a complete short form as a preliminary warm-up. The effect of these techniques is that the player is in a better state of preparedness to begin the sport or other activity, and this raises the quality of the performance, increasing the possibilities for success.

Tai chi works better than many standard warm-up exercises practiced before different sports, in that it prepares the mind as well as conditioning the body. The static exercises provide a transition between preparation and performance, clearing mental space as if preparing the mind for action. The exercises have a grounding effect, which brings the player into the heart of the moment. This has the effect of improving the ability to focus.

These pages give just a handful of examples to show how tai chi can enhance enjoyment and performance in the different sports, but the contribution it can make to performance in activities as wide-ranging as dance and other stage arts, chess, and other activities that require mental concentration, has yet to be explored.

ROCK-CLIMBING

Success in rock-climbing is linked directly to the ability to relax in difficult situations. This is studied closely in pushing hands. Climbers who also practice tai chi report that their balance and ease of movement is improved by tai chi, and these are valuable skills on the rock face.

HORSERIDING

In tai chi and in horse-riding there is a need to feel through the whole body, from head to toe, and riders have noticed that tai chi raises their body awareness, so that they are able to center through the horse. When correctly seated they feel the top of their head relate to their seat in the saddle and their feet in the stirrups, so that they

Because tai chi exercises the body as a whole and tones up the mind, it makes an excellent preparation for any sport.

In a relationship between a person and an animal, the body energies
of the two interact. This provides the opportunity to explore new forms
of communication.

earth through the horse. This posture creates the conditions for good communication with the animal. Partner training in tai chi naturally heightens a rider's awareness of the relationship with the horse. The qualities of listening and sticking, important in tai chi, are experienced through contact with the horse's mouth through the reins, as well as through the sitting posture. It is significant that the quality called joining in tai chi is mirrored by the quality called join up by the internationally famous trainer, Monty Roberts.

RACKET SPORTS

The development of whole body energy in tai chi (see pages 28-9) develops an understanding of how to use relaxed power. Tai chi works on the principle that the force of the whole body is far greater than that of an isolated limb movement, and it works to develop this force. People who play racket sports, such as tennis and squash, find that with the help of tai chi their strokes become more powerful with seemingly less physical effort.

GOLF

Better coordination is one of the effects of tai chi. Ability in many sports depends on good coordination. Success in golf relies on excellent coordination to make a perfect swing, so improved body coordination effected through tai chi can enormously improve one's handicap.

TEAM SPORTS

Gathering energy inward and channeling it to wherever it is needed is fundamental to tai chi. Learning how to manage and conserve energy through tai chi practice increases stamina, improves teamwork, and so enhances quality playing time in team sports and games, such as baseball and soccer, basketball and ice hockey.

The quality of a golf swing may improve as a result of improved concentration and better coordination developed during tai chi practice.

7

TAI CHI
EXPERIENCES

ACHIEVING SELF-FULFILMENT

What many beginners enjoy most about tai chi is the wonderfully relaxed way they feel after practice. Tai chi exercises the body but does not strain it, and although it uses energy, it also regenerates it, so people rarely feel exhausted after a class. As they progress, however, some encounter difficulties with physical aspects of tai chi, such as balance, emotional restrictions, or resistance to working with a partner in pushing hands. Challenging these impediments to progress is the essence of the art, for beginning tai chi means setting out on a journey toward greater self-fulfilment and deeper relationships with others.

It is simple things, such as walking, that people find difficult when they begin tai chi. In fact practice brings home to newcomers how complex the action of walking really is. During the first weeks it is a good idea to practice slowly moving from one step to another, getting used to the way it feels when the weight changes. This can cause aching legs at first, because when the tai chi movements are performed properly, the body's center of gravity stays very low and the legs work harder than they usually do. It really feels as if they are carrying the weight of the whole body.

One of the aims of tai chi is to restore to the adult body the flexibility it enjoyed in infancy.

Ease of movement is tied to good balance, and their balance is something many adults have not tested since childhood. Some people do not realize how much their balance has deteriorated over the years. People sometimes begin simply by steadying themselves with one hand against a wall and lifting just one heel off the floor. Once they feel comfortable with that, they practice lifting the foot an inch from the ground for a few seconds. In time, the leg muscles strengthen and the sense of balance improves so it becomes possible to stand on one leg and bend the other knee for a minute or more.

Tai chi cultivates ease of movement, something modern lifestyle inhibits. We sit on chairs and are carried by escalators. We can almost get away without moving. One of the aims of tai chi is to restore some of the wonderful flexibility of movement children naturally have. The next two pages show how tai chi can encourage children to retain much of their natural mobility into adulthood. Adults, by contrast, need to work at loosening up. Practicing journeying from lying on the floor to sitting and then to standing, in a smooth, gradual, unbroken sequence of movements is a good way of overcoming resistance to movement. Another is to squat for a minute or two now and again. Squatting opens the ankle joints, stretches the Achilles tendon, and mobilizes the hip joints.

Emotional blocks sometimes prevent us from moving freely. Western men have tended to be especially inhibited. Although society is changing rapidly, men still tend to be competitive and overaggressive, or to have lost their sense of warrior spirit. Modern men are more open to a different type of strength based on intelligence and flexibility. Tai chi shows them how to redress the imbalances caused by overcompensation, find a balance, and become a new kind of "gentle man."

Women rarely know their own strength. They are often not in touch with it. Many are afraid to find it, because to do so can be shocking. By developing their awareness, through practicing tai chi, women can access their warrior energy. Practicing the punch is one way of doing this. Just making a fist

Squatting is a good way of getting a feel for balance.

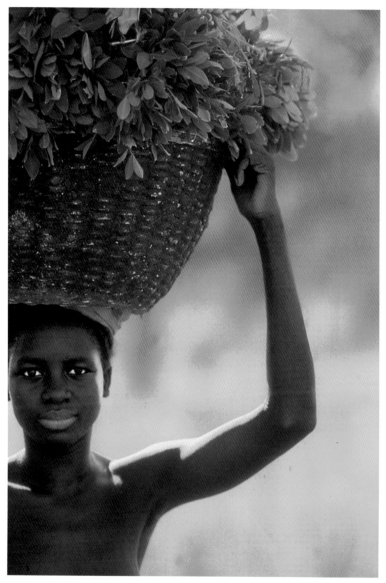

CARING FOR THE FEET

The feet are undeservedly neglected considering how much we depend on them. They need lots of attention. Tai chi raises the awareness of the feet through grounding and earthing exercises, as well as movement. They benefit from being massaged after washing at least once a day, as shown on page 25.

Cultural differences are evident in the way people move. Men and women in Asian, West Indian, and African societies often move more gracefully than Westerners. In tribal societies, some people retain their natural flexibility and sense of balance simply because from childhood they learn to balance heavy objects on the head.

and considering how it feels can bring to the surface a process that is going on beneath. Exercises like this put women in touch with a new part of themselves.

In many ways, tai chi is an exacting discipline. Executing several complex movements simultaneously demands perfect concentration. Learners are sometimes surprised to encounter an internal resistance to learning the form which may manifest itself by repeating the same mistake over and over again. One way of overcoming this is to take notes in class and practice at home; another is to visualize the resistance as a bung, stopping the flow of life energy like a cork stops bubbles escaping from a bottle of champagne. Equally, however, it is important to check one's motivation for taking up tai chi. Giving into urging from strong-minded friends who know what is best ("You should do tai chi") can leave people in an unconscious state of resentment which can surface as some form of resistance or mental block when they practice.

The following pages present the personal accounts of some people who practice tai chi today. Their stories are very different, but one thing they all show is that when it comes to tai chi, what counts is personal motivation. There is only one reason for taking it up and one reason for continuing with it, and that is that it benefits your body and your mind.

Dancing is one activity in Western society in which rhythm and graceful movement have an accepted place.

GROWING AND CHANGING

Stiff-limbed, inflexible-minded adult tai-chi learners have to work at regaining some of the softness and flexibility of their childhood bodies, and their youthful spontaneity. Children play unaffectedly, express their emotions uninhibitedly, and indulge their natural creativity and other abilities unselfconsciously. Why, then, would they need tai chi? Change – a key theme of childhood – may be part of the answer. Physically, mentally, and emotionally children grow up with change as a part of their everyday experience. Tai chi movements can give them an inner stability.

There was a time, not so long ago, when children of the great tai chi families were made to learn the art from as early as five years. They were, after all, the ones who would be carrying the lineage. To have to learn the disciplines of the tai chi form at such an age must have been extremely difficult for them. Enforced learning of a form is a burden for a child of any age, and it could be dangerous in that it might crush a wild young spirit.

Tai chi is unsuitable for a child as young as five, but can provide a way of channeling the natural enthusiasm for play of older children. Their approach to playing with the principles of tai chi should be an inspiration for any adult. Based as it is on the concept of yin-yang or polarity of opposites, tai chi offers endless possibilities for exploring movement. Children have fun investigating the movement potential of concepts such as large and small, loud and quiet, round and sharp, light and heavy. Most are in touch

with the imagination and able to access qualities in their bodies through visualization.

Every individual is different, but I have noticed through working with children that certain age groups seem to have particular needs, and tai chi seems to benefit children in the pre-adolescent years especially. It seems to help them establish a solidity and develop a sense of self.

Bodies differ, especially when they are still growing, but there seems to be a shift in emphasis around the age of eight. Children of that age group still love to act out being wild, ferocious, or still, but they are beginning to want to try some of the postures from the form and wrangle with the structure and discipline that goes with them. When taught a short sequence they respond well to a chance to express their creativity. One class had fun renaming the postures up to Single Whip, coming up with wonderful ideas. Duckfeet, Zombie, Rolling Waves, and Fat Horse seemed far better descriptions than the original names for the movements their bodies were making.

During the often dramatic teen years tai chi can act as an anchor, enabling young people to retain a solid sense of self while beginning to venture outward into the world and into new relations with other people. Teenagers tend to want to fool around physically, pushing and shoving each other. Through Pushing Hands they can channel their physical energy,

HIGH AS A MOUNTAIN

"Be as still as a mountain and move like a great river" is a classic tai chi saying. When they become the mountain, children are learning to feel grounding and rooting. They begin to see how the shape of their body works and to feel it in the strongest way. When they become a river, they learn what freedom in movement feels like. Exercises like this enable children to learn the form through experience rather than via the imposed study of theory.

HOLDING A STANCE

Children display much greater flexibility than adults and their bodies are softer. It is important not to strain young bones, joints, ligaments, tendons, and muscles. They are still growing right into their late teenage years. Whereas in adult tai chi the emphasis is often on holding a posture to develop stamina or build strength, children and teenagers must never do this. It can put strain on a young body and to stress a limb, or the spine, neck, or pelvis of someone who is still growing can be damaging.

developing a familiarity with touch. Thinking about the principles underlying the practice can give them an angle on the often confusing realms of interaction with other people, and a philosophy for dealing with them.

In the West, there are still too few children's tai chi classes. Yet once the benefits of tai chi for older children especially are explained to families, the response is often enthusiastic, and the result – a tai chi family.

TAI CHI EXPERIENCES

The following six pages present the stories of fourteen people who have incorporated tai chi into their lives. They are people of varying ages and backgrounds. For some, their journey into tai chi began only recently, and for others, tai chi has been a regular part of their lives for years. What these diverse tai chi students have in common is that all have benefited from their practice of the art. Here, they explain the different ways in which tai chi has enriched their lives.

ALISON FORD
AGE: **21**
SOCIAL WORKER
BEGAN TAI CHI:
SIX MONTHS AGO

While she was taking her graduation examinations at college, Alison looked for something to ease the stress. Her mental tension was interwoven with emotional unease because she felt depressed. She wanted to slow down inside her head and find a sense of direction in her life. She was drawn to qigung, which helped but did not fully meet her needs.

After leaving college Alison took up tai chi. She tried out different teachers and knew immediately when she found the right one. Now she has a renewed enthusiasm for life, and brings a different approach to it. Tai chi, she feels, has brought the change about. Rather than worry and try to work things out in her head, she now feels her way with decisions, and this, she says, is because tai chi has awoken a new sensitivity in her body. Alison's approach to life is now happier. Recently, the value of tai chi has been recognized by her superiors at work, who have sponsored a ten-week tai chi course for her to take place at work.

And tai chi has had another important and unforeseen effect on her inner life. It has put Alison in touch with a need to express herself which she had never recognized. At first she experienced it as an uncomfortable physical sensation in her chest and throat whenever she practiced. Encouraged by her teacher, she is beginning to express herself through drawing, and rekindling her love of singing, discovering, in the process, an exciting new world.

HARRY GOLDSTEIN
AGE: **67**
RETIRED, FORMER BUSINESS MANAGER
BEGAN TAI CHI:
2 YEARS AGO

Wanting to maintain a good level of health and fitness, and able to spend more time on himself, Harry has been enjoying tai chi since he retired. It was the need for exercise that first brought him to a class, but he now finds that what he values most is a new ability to relax in potentially stressful situations. He has developed greater tolerance of others. He is more aware of himself in relation to those around him and finds it easier to respond positively. His reactions have sharpened up, he has noticed, and he is generally more alert mentally. His enthusiasm for the art is bestowing rich returns.

Harry is surprised to find himself less physically inhibited than he was before starting tai chi. He has noticed a change in his body's capacity to heal after injury. Knocks, bumps, and one fall in particular have cleared up more quickly than has been his experience in the past.

SONNY FREEMAN
AGE: **13**
SCHOOL STUDENT
BEGAN TAI CHI:
6 WEEKS AGO

CARLA FREEMAN
AGE: **47**
HOUSEWIFE,
SONNY'S MOTHER
BEGAN TAI CHI:
6 WEEKS AGO

Some time before Sonny and his mother Carla joined a weekly tai chi class, Sonny had been looking for something he could do to build up his confidence and self-esteem. He was being bullied at school. He is big for his age, but he is not like the other kids, bunking off school and hanging around. At first, seeking to develop his personal power, he tried aikido, but he later realized it was not really giving him what he needed. He was attracted to tai chi and found a local class, but because it was an adults' class, he had to nudge his mother into joining so he could accompany her.

Sonny's ideas of what he might achieve were realistic, he was not expecting tai chi to solve all his problems. He likes working on his own and finding things out for himself.

Sonny quickly found he was enjoying the non-combative nature of tai chi. In aikido he was always picked on to be thrown because he was bigger than his classmates. After only six weeks he is feeling more relaxed, confident, and happier. He is not such a target at school and is handling the other guys better. He thinks some of them will come round to see things his way.

And Carla is also realizing the benefits of tai chi. Her joints always used to hurt after the keep fit and aerobics classes she used to attend, and that has stopped. She is already experiencing higher energy levels, enjoying the exercise, and especially likes the manageable approach to meditation through earth-breathing, sunrise and sunset, and other movements (see pages 156–7). She feels she can listen to people better.

DONNA LOPEZ
AGE: **33**
ARTIST AND
ART TEACHER
BEGAN TAI CHI:
9 YEARS AGO

A thesis she wrote during her final year at art school, in which she explored the links between visionary art and Taoism, brought Donna in contact with tai chi. She found herself transfixed by the graceful movements and joined a class.

Soon after she began tai chi she found that only fifteen minutes' daily practice made her feel more relaxed physically while centering her mentally. This proved a great advantage, because she worked long hours into the night as a waitress to support her career as an artist. She went on to manage the restaurant and it was then that she realized how useful partnerwork can be. Through it she understood how she was relating to others, and was better able to build good relations with her staff and deal with customers' needs and demands. She had always been afraid to assert herself and has learned how to do so in a rewarding way, without dominating or being aggressive.

Over time, practicing longer stances has strengthened her legs. Her spine and pelvis have freed up and tension in the muscles of her neck and shoulders has eased. Always keen on horse-riding, she soon began to ride more lightly, to connect with the ground through her horse in a new way. She also noticed that her awareness of balance has improved. Her horse seemed happier, too, and both enjoyed more relaxed quality riding time together.

Donna's life has transformed while she has been practicing tai chi, and tai chi became an important anchor during major life changes – through the breakup of her marriage and when she left her home and job. At difficult times like these, tai chi practice keeps energy levels high and maintains health. It earths the spirit. These strengths gave Donna the courage she needed to face the changes. Since these difficult times she has always used tai chi to enable her to live her life to the full.

Today, an artist and art teacher, she calls on the philosophies of tai chi to teach her how to let go and express herself more easily. She works with a tai chi tutor, and notices how people free up to paint and draw far more quickly and easily when they are involved in tai chi movement.

ROOPI PATEL
AGE: **33**
ART STUDENT
BEGAN TAI CHI:
8 YEARS AGO

MARIA CONTI
AGE: **59**
CARES FOR HER MOTHER
BEGAN TAI CHI:
8 YEARS AGO

Maria began practicing tai chi when she was 51. She was only middle-aged, but she felt like someone much older, with stiffening ankles and lower back pain. Now she says she is stronger and more supple than when she was 30, and this has restored her confidence in her body, and renewed her sense of self-worth. When she began tai chi she was employed doing heavy kitchen work. Practice gave her a practical knowledge of her skeleton and body mechanics, and the balance and coordination that enabled her to perform these tasks with greater ease than people 20 years her junior. In time her ankles loosened up and her back pain disappeared.

Over the years she has found that her health has improved, especially her resistance to infection, and her weight has stabilized. She is more relaxed, and she feels more balanced emotionally. She can see things much more clearly, and finds happiness in everyday events. Before beginning tai chi she used to lose energy by continually looking outward for happiness. Now Maria passes her inspiration onto others, running her own classes, including some for older people.

Roopi's study of tai chi was especially beneficial during her second pregnancy. She joined a class several of her friends were attending, just because it seemed fun. After about a year she signed up for a weekend workshop, which was to be a turning point in her life. The course focused on connecting with the pelvis, and it came at a time when Roopi was making a decision about whether to advance her career or have another child. Through tai chi she realized how much anxiety and fear she held in her pelvis from the difficult birth of her first child. The postures helped her achieve a feeling of freedom and empowerment as she met her fears. The experience restored her confidence in her body and gave her an emotional clarity. She realized that in fact she wanted to have another child.

For her pregnancy, Roopi drew up a health and fitness program, and used tai chi to make herself stick to it. She gave up smoking, and every time she wanted a cigarette she performed some tai chi postures instead. As her pregnancy progressed, she became concerned that she might not be able to continue tai chi into the ninth month. Would she have the flexibility and mobility? She should not have worried, she says. As she shed her inhibitions, she enjoyed being the star of the class – though a comedy star, as she sees it, since she was well into the final stages of the tai chi sword form. She felt an enjoyable satisfaction at wielding a sword when she had a huge, pregnant stomach. She went on to have a trouble-free home birth.

CRISTINA NEILSEN
AGE: **70**
WRITER
BEGAN TAI CHI:
14 YEARS AGO

Cristina started tai chi when she was well into her fifties. She loved the flow of the movements and has enjoyed the learning process. When she began, she was worried about a pain which she thought might be the beginning of arthritis in her left knee. After a few months of careful guidance and regular practice, it had gone. Now, all signs of arthritis have disappeared. Cristina speaks of how her energy has increased with her age. She can now walk uphill easily, and she breathes better. She finds the discipline of the moves has improved her concentration and continues to maintain her mental alertness. At the same time, studying tai chi movement has given her an inner joy in free movement outside the form. It makes her more spontaneous and puts her in touch with a natural wildness in her spirit. She describes herself as a healthier and happier person than before she began tai chi.

GERALD DUPUIS
AGE: **17**
STUDYING FOR
THE
INTERNATIONAL
BACCALAUREATE
BEGAN TAI CHI:
6 WEEKS AGO

Gerald has never been attracted to team and other sports. Although he knew he could not learn a sport, he felt he needed exercise, and was looking for a form of physical recreation that would make him feel good when he came across tai chi. He has just left school and started college, so he is experiencing a challenge starting a new social life among a new set of people.

He is enjoying his first experience of tai chi immensely. He likes this way of answering his needs for physical exercise, especially its non-competitive nature. The way of tai chi is already unfolding for him in exciting ways. For example, he is experiencing new physical sensations in his feet, and is enthusiastically exploring this new territory. Gerald looks upon his class as quality time for himself, a space in his life where he is free from the stresses of college and studies.

RAISA MALINSKI
AGE: **39**
COMPANY ADMINISTRATOR
BEGAN TAI CHI:
5 YEARS AGO

Having heard people talk about tai chi and seen a little of it here and there, Raisa eventually took it up. Over the last five years it has become an important part of her life. She has noticed marked changes slowly taking place in her physical condition. She has noticed marked improvements in her balance and coordination, she is more supple, and her circulation is better. She has a longer back than normal which has caused outbreaks of back pain and she is regularly treated by an osteopath, who has noted a steady improvement. She tends to suffer from asthma, which has eased considerably and she no longer needs daily medication for it.

But, she reports, the greatest gift that tai chi has given her is the ability to manage her difficulties better. Raisa used to find it hard to cope with the stress and anxiety caused by long hours working at a demanding job. The philosophy of tai chi has enabled her to accept who she is, to feel well grounded, and to move steadily toward her goals, both personal and work-related. This has given her a sense of space. Her perception of life has broadened. Raisa is now easier on herself, calmer, and more cheerful, and she attributes this rise in the quality of her life to her eternally evolving practice of tai chi.

TAYO OLUGBO
AGE: **34**
PERFORMER
BEGAN TAI CHI:
15 YEARS AGO

Brought up in a rough city district, Tayo had to develop a tough facade in order to survive. He has a Nigerian heritage, so he needed to deal with racist attitudes as part of his growing up. He had a fiery temper and he took up kung fu to find a way of channeling it, as well as learning to look after himself. He honoured Bruce Lee as The Great One.

Tayo is big, strong, and fast, but inside, he found all this energy he was generating frightening. When he moved to a college in a smaller town, he began to look for something to replace kung fu. He had always been attracted to the old wise man in the kung fu movies who seemed so relaxed, happy, and in command of his situation. At college he found tai chi, and with his martial background he could see the links between the disciplined energy of kung fu and the relaxed movements of tai chi. He tried it out, but soon became bored with having to rework things over and again in class.

Then something happened that was to hook him. During his teen years Tayo had learned to love basketball and was playing regularly in a major league. After his move to another town he was accepted to play for the city team, which upgraded him to the national league. One thing bothered him – a painful knee was restricting his play. Yet after only three months of tai chi practice he noticed that his knee problem had disappeared. He was now using his frame differently as a result of the tai chi practice. Seeing that tai chi really worked convinced Tayo to continue his training. In time, he calmed down enough to be able to discover more about the mental aspects of the art, in particular the quality of stillness. This is now at the hub of his continuing study of tai chi.

AMY CHANDLER
AGE: **48**
SOLICITOR
BEGAN TAI CHI:
2 YEARS AGO

Amy happened to encounter tai chi at just the right time in her life. She was on vacation in Greece at a center for holistic studies, and looking for direction. Her 25-year marriage had just ended and, moreover, she was coming to terms with a second hip replacement. She felt awkward, even disabled, and this affected her confidence and sense of self-worth. She was afraid to face the reality of her new body and she had an aversion to touch. She was also experiencing the numbing effects of painkilling drugs. She described herself as somehow having lost a vital connection.

It was during her vacation that Amy was introduced to tai chi. Its effects were inspiring. She immediately sensed that her mind and body were reconnecting and this made her feel as if she had been released from a prison sentence. The experience inspired her to continue with tai chi back home. Having found a way to meet her difficulties, she is now far more aware, mentally and physically, feels energized and more alive, and has found strength and happiness.

ALAN MCPHERSON
AGE: **39**
SCHOOL TEACHER
BEGAN TAI CHI:
8 YEARS AGO

BENJAMIN CHAN
AGE: **35**
PRIMARY SCHOOL TEACHER
BEGAN TAI CHI:
9 YEARS AGO

Ben was looking for direction in his life and had found nothing to satisfy his quest. He is a natural seeker, but his efforts had led to nothing. He had reached the point of disillusionment and this kept him in a state of depression. Rather than read another book that left him with more questions than answers, he decided to have one more try, but this time to channel his efforts in another direction. He now he explored a path he had not tried before, and joined a tai chi class.

At last, Ben quickly discovered that this new journey into his body was beginning to deliver the kind of satisfaction he had looked for with such perseverance. He found that tai chi lifted his depression, and his disparate studies began to merge into an enlightening physical experience. Tai chi, Ben says, has taught him to trust in himself, in life, and in what life has to offer. The greater flexibility of his body, gradually brought about through tai chi, has been matched by an increased adaptability in his attitude to life. Today, Ben is a person with a renewed and infectious enthusiasm for life.

Alan came across a local tai chi class, and joined partly from curiosity and partly from a desire to develop a healthier relationship with his body. He had a new job in which he was supervising teenagers at a field studies center and he needed to improve his strength and stamina.

The tai chi classes helped him physically and were enjoyable, but they left him feeling unfulfilled, mainly, he felt, because he was not particularly interested in their strongly martial approach. He did enjoy learning a stick form, however. On a whim he attended a short course that combined tai chi with personal development and experience of nature. This resonated with him and he began learning with the new teacher.

Tai chi has raised his consciousness, he says, and changed his awareness. He experiences life differently now. Simply standing on the earth has a fuller and richer dimension because he is so much more aware of the earth beneath his feet, the air around him, and the sky above his head. He finds the tai chi training especially relevant in his work as a teacher, where he spends a large proportion of his time outdoors, and he has benefited from improved health and resistance to illness. Through experiencing the links between his inner self and his awareness of his environment, Alan finds he can encourage his young students to expand their awareness.

STYLES AND SCHOOLS

Although there is only a handful of principal styles of tai chi, each style has many variations, and each variation has many approaches. Deciding what style to learn could therefore be a difficult decision. Pages 22–23 explain the origins of the different tai chi styles and trace the development of some of their variations and versions. These pages give more information about how these styles and their variations differ.

CHOOSING A STYLE

In tai chi, as in any art or discipline, people who teach or practice may support a particular style or practice wholeheartedly, sometimes even denying the validity of other styles. Tai chi teachers can be found who deny the martial applications of the art, arguing that tai chi is purely a system of exercises. It is advisable not to heed such partisan approaches. Essentially, tai chi is neither health nor self-defense – it is all and both of these things. More importantly it is about the development of the whole person: body, mind, and spirit.

Naturally there are arguments for and against each style and each variation, but the similarities between the styles are often more striking, and it is important to realize that the current tendency toward polarization of styles is not how it has always been. The founders of the Yang, Wu and Hou styles (see page 22) all began by simply studying tai chi. Later, far from indulging in bitter rivalry, they established a tradition of learning in an atmosphere of collective respect for one another and for their art, which was essentially the application of the yin-yang theory to martial arts. Their intelligence and humility resulted in the collective development of tai chi (see box opposite).

The 20th century saw the spread of tai chi westward, beyond the borders of China. One of the key figures in this dissemination is Cheng Man-ch'ing, who studied Yang style under its founder's grandson. Cheng Man-ch'ing altered the Yang Big Form, which had been developed by his teacher, to create a Short Form. After the 1960s this concise version of the Yang form became popular worldwide. Yet Cheng Man-ch'ing did not, perhaps, set out to create a new style. He did not think of his Short Form of 37 postures as more simple than his teacher's 108-posture Big Form. He developed it as a way of pulling together the essential elements of the art, and in doing this he presented a different way of practicing which was accessible to a wider range of people.

FINDING A CLASS

Tai chi is very widespread in Western countries, so it should be possible for most people to find a weekly local class, although not necessarily in the style you particularly want to learn. Remember that it does not matter which style you learn. All are expressions of tai chi. Join the class and learn the style with goodwill. If you later go on to learn a second style, you will find it useful and interesting to have had the experience of learning a different approach.

However, if you live in a town or a suburb you may have a bewildering choice. A tai chi class on the south side of the street may look like a different art from the one happening on the north side, and there may be another around the corner. If you are drawn to a certain style, there is no reason why you should not join a class where it is taught. But do not close your mind to other approaches. A more important consideration than style when choosing a class is to find a good environment in which to learn. If you have a choice, try to find a teacher with whom you feel you can make progress, regardless of which school or variation they teach.

If it is difficult for you to get to a regular class, look for tai chi courses. Perhaps you can get away for a weekend or holiday at a center where tai chi is taught. With the help of this book and perhaps a video you will still be able to practice regularly. Maybe you can find a friend to practice with.

CLASSIC STYLES AND SCHOOLS

CHEN STYLE
Although this is regarded as the first recognized style of tai chi, it is only now becoming popular worldwide. It is characterized by dynamic, physically demanding movements that strengthen the legs and open the hips and other joints. The style clearly demonstrates a polarity of fast and slow, small and large. It is a good one to practice for anyone wishing to attain a high degree of physical strength and suppleness. It is entirely suitable for beginners.

YANG STYLE
Yang is the family name, not to be confused with the concept of yin-yang, and Yang style is perhaps the world's most popular tai chi style. It is often considered the gentlest style, which makes it immediately accessible to the elderly and the not so fit. However, practicing Yang style can result in an extremely fit and agile body. There is more than one version: Big Form (also called Longform) has more postures and takes longer to perform. Beginners usually opt for the Short Form.

CHENG MAN-CH'ING STYLE
This popular style is practiced the world over. Cheng Man-ch'ing, who was instrumental in bringing tai chi to the West, condensed and softened the longer Yang form. This style strongly emphasizes softness and relaxation, making it an especially graceful style, though no less effective as a martial art. It is the style described step by step on pages 84–143.

WU STYLE
This style, though generally called Wu style, is a small frame version of Yang style, characterized by a forward lean. ("Small frame" means that a shorter stance is adopted than in Yang style, which results in generally smaller body movements.) It is suitable for beginners and for more advanced learners.

LI (HOU) STYLE
This is the Old Wu style as it has reached us today, devised by Wu Yu-hsiang (see pages 22–3). The style is characterized by a very small frame, with a follow step (this enables you to cover

ground with a small stance, so that two or three small steps would be equal to one long stance: thus, this style gives mobility. It is not as widely taught as Yang and Cheng Man-ch'ing styles.

SUN STYLE

Sun Lu-t'ang, a master of Chinese internal martial arts, founded this style (see pages 22–3. His style is characterized by small circular movements and high stances. These train people to apply tai chi in their normal walking position, rather than lowering the stance as in a self-defense situation. Because you perform the postures in a normal walking position, you do not use energy getting into a lower stance.

MODERN STYLES AND SCHOOLS

PEKING (BEIJING) STYLE

This style, devised in the late 1940s by Master Li T'ien-shih at the request of the Wushu Council of China (see pages 22-3) is fairly widely taught. It was conceived as an accessible short form which, it was hoped, would be widely adopted and would raise the health of the Chinese people. The founders were also asked to create a standard style that would cater for the rising interest in tai chi as a competitive sport. A whole system of pushing hands was devised to accompany the sets. There is a 24-step form, in which the essential elements of Yang style are condensed. A 36-step form was created, but did not catch on. The 48-step style, which combines the essential elements of Chen, Yang, Wu, and Hou styles, is a standard competition form, and there is an 88-step form.

ASSESSING TEACHERS

People often worry about who to learn with and how to go about finding the right teacher. The best advice is: stop worrying, but be alert, and do ask questions. When you have located a class, go along early and speak to the teacher. Ask if you can watch the class, or join in.

Do not be afraid of trying out different classes with different teachers, or of asking questions. Find out from whom each teacher has learned and how long they have been studying tai chi. It may be unwise to learn with a teacher who has been studying for less than three years and considerably more than three years is the ideal.

Perhaps most important, however, is to ask the teacher to explain what the class offers—not only what style is taught but how it is organized and what happens in it. It can be helpful to be aware of the atmosphere. When you walk into a class, ask yourself whether it resonates well with you. Feel your way. If what is offered matches what you are looking for, join. If not, try others until you find the right one.

People sometimes advise looking for a teacher who belongs to a recognized body. This is sensible and is a good way of finding a teacher. However, it is most important to be alert to your personal needs. Some excellent teachers belong to no recognized body, and there are some teachers on the lists of respected tai chi organizations who may never communicate well with you. You need a teacher who inspires you.

TEACHER TRAINING

Up to now, tai chi, unlike other martial arts, has had no gradings or recognizable stages of development. Students would become teachers if and when their own teachers considered it appropriate. Now, however, new standards are evolving to ensure that tai chi instructors are capable of teaching, and specialist magazines, such as the American

publication *Tai Chi*, publish information about new developments. In the UK, a proposal is being considered to introduce a five-year teacher training syllabus, coordinated by the T'ai Chi Union of Great Britain. To prospective teachers this may seem a long training period, but it makes sense when you think that some unrecognized schools allow their teachers to set up classes after only a few weekends of training.

Even for someone who has been learning tai chi for some years, the idea of teaching may seem nerve-wracking. Good teachers are always welcome, however. If you feel drawn to teaching but rather nervous of trying, bear in mind that the best method of teaching is to forget about it. In this way you can allow your passion for the art to evolve, and enjoy the journey. If you can teach a few trial classes, it will soon become clear whether teaching is the right step for you.

COMPETITION

For many people, tai chi is a sport, with regular competitive events. In a competition people can put their solo and partner skills to the test in a potentially stressful situation. As well as offering a challenge, competitions can be valuable forums for interclub or intercultural exchange, where people who practice tai chi have an opportunity to meet and trade views, approaches, and techniques. Some schools are geared to competitive events, others are opposed to competition in tai chi, and some are neutral on the question. Their response may have some bearing on the school you choose.

INSPIRATION FROM THE PAST

Back in the early 1800s an open-hearted interchange of ideas produced the Yang, the Wu, and what would become the Hou (Li) style. Yang Lu-ch'an, who founded the Yang style; Wu Yu-seong who developed the Hou style; and Wu Ch'uan-You, founder of the Wu style, learned and practiced together in ways which greatly benefited the development of tai chi. The little-known story of this cooperation should be an inspiration to people today and should counter the growing tendency to see one style as superior to another.

From a poor peasant family and with a great enthusiasm for tai chi, the young Yang Lu-ch'an was befriended by the more prosperous Wu family and taught the art by Wu Yu-hsiang, [14 years his junior. Hearing of the high standard of the Chen family style, his youthful teacher encouraged him to find a way of studying it. The story of how Yang worked as a servant in the Chen household and became accepted as a student (see page 2) is often told. It is less well known that after 18 years of studying Chen-style tai chi, Yang, visiting his former teacher, found his skills in Pushing Hands more advanced than Wu's. In an act that even today would be regarded as one of great humility, Wu then became Yang's student.

Yang went on to link Wu's style with that of the Chen family to develop the now-renowned Yang style. In his turn, Wu went on to study with the Chen family, and later founded his own style, now called the Old Wu {Hou or Li} style. And the cooperation continued. Yang Ban-hou studied with his father and with Wu. Later, Yang's disciple, Wu Ch'uan You, developed the second Wu style. The map on page 23 shows how these major styles of tai chi evolved from a common root. This evolution took place largely because of this spirit of cooperation, and so for this reason, it is always more rewarding to look for the similarities rather than the differences between tai chi styles.

GLOSSARY

ba gua (pa kua): Literally "eight diagrams" or the eight original trigrams (q.v.) in the ancient *I Ching* or *Book of Changes*. A soft or internal martial art in which the performer practices a series of movements based on the eight diagrams laid out on the ground in an imaginary circle, usually referred to as the "ba gua diagram."

chi (ch'i, qi): Life force or, literally translated, "life energy." Ch'i originally meant "air" or "breath" (it once described the vapor from cooking cereals) and came to signify cosmic energy. Chi exists in all matter. It circulates around the bodies of living creatures, along channels or meridians (q.v.).

classics, Chinese: The earliest written works of Chinese literature, dating from the first millennium BCE. The *Wu Ching* (five classics), are: the *I Ching (Book of Changes)*, a system of divination; the *Shih Ching (Classic of Songs or Book of Odes)*, a collection of 305 poems; the *Li Chi (Book of Rites)* describing ceremonials and an ideal Confucian state; the *Shu Ching (Classic of Documents)*, containing historical records; and the *Ch'un Ch'iu (Spring and Autumn Annals)* a chronology of Lu, Confucius's native state. These and some later works are traditionally said to have been written by Confucius and are collectively called the Thirteen Confucian Classics, although they are now known to be collections of writings and sayings of many historical figures. Other classics include the chief literature of Taoism, the *Tao Te Ching (Classic of the Way and its Power)*, traditionally ascribed to Lao Tzu, and the work of Chuang-Tzu, both though to have been written down during the 200s BCE. *See also* classics, tai chi.

classics, tai chi: The canon of writings by great exponents of tai chi set down during the last millennium They are referred to as "the classics" by experts in the art of tai chi, although they do not number among the ancient Chinese classics (q.v.). They include essays and instructions to students, such as Cheng Fan-seng's *T'ai Chi Ch'uan Ch'ing*; Wang Tsung-yueh's *T'ai Chi Ch'uan Lun*; Wu Yu-hsiang's *Exposition of Insights Into The Thirteen Positions*; and Li I-yu's *Five-Character Secret*.

crown center: The seventh energy center, seated in and around the head. Also called the pai hui.

earthing: *see* grounding

form: The continuous sequence of choreographed postures which is the essence of tai chi. Each tai chi style has its own characteristic form or forms, which may differ in the postures included and the way they are performed, and in the time they take to play.

grounding: Establishing and maintaining a good connection with the earth center through the feet and the ground.

heart energy center: The fourth energy center, also called the middle tantien, located in the center of the chest.

hexagram: A group of six broken or unbroken lines or two trigrams (q.v.) which may be combined into 64 patterns.

hsingi: A Chinese soft martial art influenced by Taoist thought, in which movements take place in straight lines and the more advanced forms are based on the movements of twelve animals.

jin: Whole body energy, which may be fast or slow, light or solid, depending on what type of energy is needed. When used correctly, each part of the body contributes to a movement, so that the body works as a coordinated whole.

meridians: Hidden channels connecting all parts of the body along which chi (q.v.) travels.

mind intent: Mindset or attitude; the thought and intention governing a tai chi movement.

natural way: A fundamental concept of tai chi is to search for the way the world works naturally and to try to act accordingly. Tai chi teaches that rather than use force to try to make things happen it is better to try to find the way things work naturally and wait for the right moment to achieve the objective without force.

palm away: The palm of the hand is turned to face outward, away from the body.

palm facing: The palm of the hand faces the body.

posture: A choreographed movement in tai chi, in which several parts of the body may move simultaneously.

qigung (chigong or chi kung): A practice closely related to tai chi which works to build and move energy. Its literal translation is "energy work" and it cultivates chi (q.v.) to promote well-being and vitality by recharging the body's energy source.

root center: The hui yin, also called the base or root center because it is the first and lowest of the energy centers, seated at the base of the spine and filling the lower pelvis.

sacrum: The large bone shaped like an inverted triangle that forms the lower part of the spine and the back of the pelvic girdle. The sacrum ("sacred bone") consists of five fused vertebrae (spinal bones). It forms joints with the fifth lumbar vertebra above and the coccyx (tail bone) below. The sacro-iliac joint, between the sacrum and the pelvic girdle is securely ligamented so that the sacrum is immobile except during pregnancy.

shape: The position made by the body during a tai chi movement, or by a part of the body, such as the arms.

soft: To soften a part of the body, such as the hips, is to relax it physically and mentally. There is a strong mental component in softening which distinguishes it from physical relaxation. Tai chi is one of a number of "soft" or "internal" martial arts, in which the mind has a central role in deciding and taking action and which emphasize the gathering and utilizing of internal energy. An essential principle of the soft martial arts is that the energy of an opponent's blow is used against him or her.

solar plexus center: The third energy center, located just below the ribs, also called by its Chinese name, the chung wan.

step up: To take an adjustment step in which the back foot moves in toward the front foot.

stick: To keep two parts of the body (or two tai chi players) close, even while moving.

substantial and insubstantial: When the weight of the body rests on the right leg, the right leg is substantial and the left insubstantial, and vice-versa.

tai chi (t'ai chi): A system of exercises for health and self-development with martial applications; a soft or internal martial art; a shortened form of "t'ai chi ch'uan" (q.v.).

t'ai chi ch'uan: A Chinese soft or internal martial art. Literally translated, the term means "supreme pole fist."

tantien: This Chinese term commonly describes the second energy center, located in the lower back and extending forward to about 3 inches below the navel. It is also called the hara or sacral center. It is the lower of three tantiens. The middle tantien is the heart center (q.v.); and the upper tantien is the sixth energy center, located in the middle of the forehead and also called the third eye or brow center.

Taoism (Daoism): A major Chinese philosophy, thought to have been founded some time before the 300s BCE, which later branched out into a religion. The English word "Taoism" is used to translate two Chinese terms: *tao chia* (the school of thought of the tao (dao) or way) and *tao chiao* (The Taoist (Daoist) religion).

throat center: The fifth energy center, located at the front of the neck, also called by its Chinese name, the hsuan chi.

trigram: A group of three broken or unbroken lines; half a hexagram (q.v.).

waist: In tai chi this term refers to the lower abdomen and pelvis.

yin and yang: General terms for opposing but complementary forces of nature, the female and male principles. The terms are believed to have originally meant "shady" and "sunny" since the northern side of a mountain is termed yin in Chinese and the southern side yang. Yin and yang are the principles governing the universe, which alternate in space and time.

CHINESE TERMS

Many different systems have been devised to transliterate Chinese, a language with no alphabet and many sounds unknown in European languages, into English. Until recently, the Wade-Giles system has been commonly used in British English and the Yale system in American English. These different systems account for the confusing differences in the English spelling of Chinese words. For example, under the Wade-Giles system, "tai chi chuan" is written "t'ai chi ch'uan." The apostrophes are guides to pronunciation, indicating that the "t" in "t'ai" is pronounced closer to a "t" sound in English than to a "d," and the "ch" in "ch'uan" is pronounced closer to an English "j" sound than a "ch."

In 1958 the Chinese government officially sanctioned a new system, called pinyin. This is now widely taught and extensively used by the media, both in China and in the West. In pinyin "tai chi chuan" is written "taijiquan;" "ch'i" is written "qi," "tao" and "Taoism" are written "dao" and "Daoism," and so on. The official adoption of the pinyin system explains why we now write "Mao Zedong" and "Beijing" instead of "Mao Tse-tung" or "Mao Tse Tung" and "Peking."

It will be many years, however, before pinyin becomes universally adopted and in this book we have used the spelling which seems most widely understood, so we use 'tai chi' instead of the now official 'daiji'; Taoism instead of Daoism, chi instead of ch'i or qi, and so on. For less well-known words, however, we have adopted the modern spelling, so that chi gung (Yale system) or chi kung (Wade-Giles) is written as qigung (pinyin). Where we felt clarification might be needed we have occasionally inserted the pinyin spelling in parentheses after the old spelling. The names of people who became well known before the 1950s are spelled in the old way.

USEFUL ADDRESSES

EUROPE
Taijiquan and Qigong Federation
for Europe
Web: www.taijiquan-qigung.com

FRANCE
Fédération Française des Tai Chi
Chuan Traditionnels
78 Rue Saint Honoré,
75001 Paris.
Tel: 01 45 43 03 96

THE NETHERLANDS
Pierre de Cat
Postbus 2271800,
AE Alcmaar.
Email: mailing@taijiquan-
qigong.com

Stichting Taijiquan Nederland
Postbus 13 26 4, 3507 LG
Utrecht.
Tel: 030 289 6336.
Publishers of Nieuwsbrief
magazine.

UK
Angus Clark – School of Living
Movement
Courses and classes in the UK
and worldwide.
+44 [0] 1647 231477
angusclark.livingmovement@
appleonline.net

Alan Peck – Natural Way Tai Chi
School
c/o Lam Rim Centre,
12 Victoria Place,
Bedminster,
Bristol 3.

Tai Chi Union for Great Britain
69 Kilpatrick Gardens,
Clarkston,
Glasgow G76 7RF.
Tel: +44 [0] 141 621 1220
Email: taichi@dial.pipex.com
Publishers of T'ai Chi Ch'uan
magazine.

USA
Universal Tai Chi Chuan
Association
Contact: Ben Lo
2901 Clement Street,
San Francisco,
CA 94121.
William Chen
2 Washington Square Village
#10J, New York,
N Y10012.
Tel: [212] 675 2816

Yang's Martial Arts Association
Contact: Dr. Yang Jwing Ming
28 Hyde Park Avenue,
Jamaica Plain,
MA 02130-4132.
Tel: [1-617] 524 8892

TAI CHI MAGAZINES
These magazines give useful
information about developments
and activities in the tai chi world,
provide interesting reading, and
are the best way to find classes,
teachers and other contacts.

Journal of Asian Martial Arts
Media Publishing Co,
821 West 24th Street,
Erie, PA 16502, USA.
Email: info@goviamedia.com
Web: www.goviamedia.com

Nieuwsbrief
published by Stichting Taijiquan
Nederland

Qi – The Journal of Traditional
Eastern Health and Fitness
Insight Graphics Inc,
Box 18476, Anaheim Hills,
CA 92817, USA.
Web: www.qi-journal.com

Qi Magazine
PO Box 116,
Manchester M20 3YN, UK.
Web: www.qimagazine.com

Tai Chi – The Leading
International Magazine of
Tai Chi Chuan
Wayfarer Publications,
2601 Siver Ridge Avenue,
Los Angeles,
CA 90039, USA.
Web: www.tai-chi.com

Tai Chi and Alternative Health
PO Box 6404,
London E18 1 EX, UK.
Tel: +44[0] 20 8502 9307

T'ai Chi Ch'uan
published by the Tai Chi Union
for Great Britain

Tai Chi International
St Vincent's Publishing,
PO Box 460,
Thorney, Peterborough,
Cambridgeshire PE6 0TQ, UK
Tel: [01733] 270 072
Email: tcinter@easynet.co.uk

Tai Chi Magazine
published by the Fédération
Française des Tai Chi Chuan
Traditionnels

**HOLISTIC
VACATIONS / RETREATS**
These three centers regularly offer
tai chi in their programs. All are
located in Europe but have an
international reputation.

Skyros, Greece
Tel: +44 [0] 171 267 4424
Email: Skyros@easynet.co.uk
Web: www.skyros.com

La Serrania, Mallorca, Spain
Tel: +34 639 306 432
Fax: +34 971 182 144

Cortijo Romero, Spain
Email: bookings@cortijo-
romero.co.uk
Web: www.cortijo-romero.co.uk

FURTHER READING

TAI CHI

Chen Wei-ming *Tai Chi Chuan Ta Wen (Questions and Answers on Tai Chi Chuan)*, translated by Ben Lo and Robert Smith, North Atlantic Books, 1985.

Cheng Man-ch'ing *Cheng Tzu's Thirteen Treatises on Tai Chi Chuan*, translated by Ben Lo and Martin Inn, North Atlantic Books, 1993.

Cheng Man-ch'ing *T'ai Chi Ch'uan*, North Atlantic Books, 1993.

Crompton, Paul *The Elements of Tai Chi*, Element Books, 1990.

Docherty, Dan *Complete T'ai Chi Ch'uan*, Crowood Press, 1997.

Lo, Benjamin *The Essence of Tai Chi Chuan: The Literary Tradition*, North Atlantic Books, 1993.

Peck, Alan *T'ai Chi: The Essential Introductory Guide*, Vermilion, 1999.

Sutton, Nigel *Applied T'ai Chi Ch'uan*, A & C Black, 1991.

Cheng Man-ch'ing *Advanced Tai Chi Form Instructions*, translated by Douglas Wile, Sweet Chi Press, New York, 1989.

In Chinese:
Yang Cheng-fu *Yang-style T'ai Chi Ch'uan* (recorded by his disciples), Taiping Book Co., Hong Kong, 1976.

Zhang San-feng *The Secret of Training, the Internal Elixir of the Taiji Art*. Preserved by Taiyi Shanren. Reprinted from ancient text by Anhua Publications, Hong Kong.

MARTIAL ARTS

Finn, Michael *Martial Arts: A Complete Illustrated History*, Stanley Paul, 1988. Available from Elite Martial Academy, 17A Filmer Road, London SW6 7BU, UK.

Wing, R.L. (Ed) *The Art of Strategy*, Thorsons, London, and Doubleday & Co, USA, 1998.

QIGUNG

Frantzis, Bruce Kumar *Opening the Energy Gates of Your Body*, North Atlantic Books, 1997.

CHINESE PHILOSOPHY AND DAOISM

Fung Yu-lan *A Short History of Chinese Philosophy*, The Free Press, 1995.

Lao Tzu Tao *Te Ching*, translated by D.C. Lau, Penguin Books, 1998.

Lao Tzu Tao *Te Ching*, translated by Richard Wilhelm, Arkana, 1998.

Lao Tzu Tao Te Ching, translated by M.H. Kwok et al, Element Books, 1998.

Wilhelm, Richard (rendered into English by Cary F. Baynes) *I Ching*, Arkana, 1999.

Wing, *R.L. The Illustrated I Ching*, Aquarian Press, 1987. A recent translation, very readable.

HEALING

Anodea, Judith *Wheels of Life, A User's Guide to the Chakra System*, Llewellyn Publications, 1990.

Mitchell, Stewart *Naturopathy – Understanding the Healing Power of Nature*, Element Books, 1998.

PICTURE CREDITS

Anglo Australian Observatory/David Malin: 15b; Barbara Richter: 84tl; Bridgeman Art Library: 20b, 55tr; Camera Press: 166t; Mary Evans Picture Library: 19bl, 161, 186bl; Fortean Picture Library: 146tl; Hutchison Library: 11, 20t, 46t, 61b, 152b, 155, 161; Image Bank: 44tl, 53br, 147t, 152t, 175tl; Images Colour Library: 19t, 148b, 170l, 171t; Journal Für Die Frau: 156; Science Photo Library: 55br; Tony Stone Images: 8cr, 22, 28t, 32tl, br, 33t, 36t, 53tr, 62tl, 148t, 150t, b, 168t, 169t, 175br.

INDEX

INDEX

INDEX